Field Epidemiology

Field Epidemiology

Edited by
MICHAEL B. GREGG

Associate Editors
Richard C. Dicker
Richard A. Goodman

New York   Oxford
OXFORD UNIVERSITY PRESS
1996

Oxford University Press

Oxford   New York
Athens   Auckland   Bangkok   Bombay
Calcutta   Cape Town   Dar es Salaam   Delhi
Florence   Hong Kong   Istanbul   Karachi
Kuala Lumpur   Madras   Madrid   Melbourne
Mexico City   Nairobi   Paris   Singapore
Taipei   Tokyo   Toronto

and associated companies in
Berlin   Ibadan

Published by Oxford University Press, Inc.,
198 Madison Avenue, New York, New York 10016

Oxford is a registered trademark of Oxford University Press

Library of Congress Cataloging-in-Publication Data
Field epidemiology / edited by Michael B. Gregg ; associate editors,
Richard C. Dicker, Richard A. Goodman.
p.   cm.
Includes bibliographical references and index.
ISBN 0-19-507207-3
1. Clinical epidemiology—Handbooks, manuals, etc.   I. Gregg,
Michael B.   II. Dicker, Richard C.   III. Goodman, Richard A.
(Richard Alan), 1949–
[DNLM: 1. Disease Outbreaks—handbooks.   2. Epidemiologic Methods—
handbooks.   3. Epidemiology—organization & administration—
handbooks.   WA 39 F453 1996]
RA652.2.C55F53   1996
614.4—dc20
DNLM/DLC
for Library of Congress   95-30843

9 8 7 6 5 4 3 2 1

Printed in the United States of America
on acid-free paper

This book is dedicated to the memory of

Alexander D. Langmuir,

originator, teacher, and practitioner of field epidemiology,
whose wisdom, vision, and inspiration have profoundly
strengthened the practice of public health
throughout the world.

PREFACE

Carl W. Tyler, Jr.

Epidemiology is becoming increasingly complex, theoretical, and specialized. While many epidemiologists are still engaged in the investigation of infectious disease problems, others are addressing new challenges such as homicides and unplanned pregnancy. Computers make it practical to calculate in seconds what might otherwise take months to complete. Whole new textbooks have appeared in such areas as pharmacoepidemiology, perinatal epidemiology, and occupational epidemiology.

Because of the advances in the real world of contemporary health problems, there is a need for a clearly written, highly usable book devoted to field epidemiology—the timely use of epidemiology in solving public health problems. This process involves the application of basic epidemiologic principles in real time, place, and person to solve health problems of an urgent or emergency nature.

This book, intended to meet this need, is based upon both science and experience. It deals with real problems, real places, and real people: nature's experiments, if you will, rather than carefully designed studies in a laboratory or clinical setting. So, in the lexicon of the epidemiologist, the book will be addressing issues relating to observational—not experimental—epidemiology.

To a great extent, this book takes it roots from the experience of the Centers for Disease Control and Prevention (CDC) over more than forty years of training health professionals in the science and art of field epidemiology. In 1951, Alexander D. Langmuir, M.D., CDC's chief epidemiologist, founded the Epidemic Intelligence

Service (EIS) and its 2-year on-the-job training program in practical, applied epidemiology. On call 24 hours a day, the trainee, called an EIS officer, has been available upon request to go into the field to help state and local health officials investigate urgent health problems. Before going into the field, however, EIS officers receive training at CDC in basic epidemiology, biostatistics, and public health practice. The 3-week, 8-hour-a-day course is designed to equip them with the essentials of how to mount a field investigation, how to investigate an epidemic, how to start a surveillance system, and how to apply science, technology, and common sense to meet real-life problems at the grass-roots level of experience.

Based on the collective experience of EIS officers and their CDC mentors, this book thus attempts to describe the relevant and appropriate operations necessary to solve urgent health problems at local, state, provincial, federal, and international levels.

Section I contains a definition of field epidemiology and only a brief review of epidemiologic principles and methods, under the assumption that the reader has some knowledge of basic epidemiologic methods. It follows with a discussion of the concepts of surveillance, particularly as they pertain to field epidmiology.

Section II covers the components of field epidemiology: (1) operational aspects of field investigations; (2) conducting a field investigation—a practical step-by-step description of what to do in the field; (3) describing the data—the elements of time, place, and person; (4) designing studies; (5) analyzing and interpreting data; (6) developing interventions; and (7) communicating the findings.

Section III covers special issues such as (1) surveys and sampling; (2) use of microcomputers in the field; (3) dealing with the public and the press; (4) legal aspects of field investigations; (5) field investigations in institutional, day care, and international settings; and (6) the collection and handling of laboratory specimens in association with a field investigation.

Copies of this book should be found more often in the briefcases of field epidemiologists than on the shelves of libraries. It is intended to be a close companion during the preparation and conduct of field investigations; it should be helpful during data analysis; and it should be a ready reference when the final epidemiologic report is being written. It is not intended to replace the detailed, specialized reference works found on the shelves of libraries in medical centers and schools of public health. Rather, it is meant to be readily accessible and to serve as an important tool for any health professional responsible for investigating epidemiologic problems.

Acknowledgments

The editors wish to express their sincere thanks to Jean M. Heslin for her dedicated and expert administrative and secretarial services, and to Sandra W. Bowden, C.P.S., for technical assistance in the preparation of this book. Our thanks, also, go to R. Elliott Churchill, M.A., for her editorial contributions.

CONTENTS

III   Special Considerations

CONTRIBUTORS

JAMES W. BUEHLER, M.D.
Associate Director, Division of HIV/
AIDS, National Center for Infectious Diseases, Centers for Disease
Control and Prevention, Atlanta,
Georgia

BRUCE B. DAN, M.D.
Executive Editor and Executive Vice
President, Medical News Network,
New York, New York

ANDREW G. DEAN, M.D., M.P.H.
Chief, Systems Development and
Support Branch, Division of
Surveillance and Epidemiology,
Epidemiology Program Office,
Centers for Disease Control and
Prevention, Atlanta, Georgia

RICHARD C. DICKER, M.D., M.Sc.
Chief, Epidemiology Training
Activity, Division of Training,
Epidemiology Program Office,
Centers for Disease Control
and Prevention, Atlanta, Georgia

STANLEY O. FOSTER, M.D., M.P.H.
Visiting Professor, International
Health, Emory University School
of Public Health, Atlanta, Georgia

RICHARD A. GOODMAN, M.D., M.P.H.
Editor, *Morbidity and Mortality
Weekly Report Series*, and Assistant Director, Epidemiology
Program Office, Centers for
Disease Control and Prevention,
Atlanta, Georgia

MICHAEL B. GREGG, M.D.
Consultant in Epidemiology,
    Epidemiologic Training, and Disease
    Surveillance, Guilford, Vermont

ROBERT A. GUNN, M.D., M.P.H.
Medical Epidemiologist, Division of
    STD/HIV, National Center for
    Prevention Services, Centers for
    Disease Control and Prevention,
    Atlanta, Georgia

WILLIAM R. JARVIS, M.D.
Chief, Investigation and Prevention
    Branch, Hospital Infections Program,
    National Center for Infectious
    Diseases, Centers for Disease Control
    and Prevention, Atlanta, Georgia

JEFFREY P. KOPLAN, M.D., M.P.H.
Executive Vice President and Director,
    The Prudential Center for Health
    Care Research, Atlanta, Georgia

WILLIAM J. MARTONE, M.D.
Director, Hospital Infections Program,
    National Center for Infectious
    Diseases, Centers for Disease Control
    and Prevention, Atlanta, Georgia

JANET MOHLE-BOETANI, M.D.
Medical Epidemiologist, Disease
    Control and Prevention Division,
    Santa Clara County Health Depart-
    ment, San Jose, California

VERLA J. NESLUND, J.D.
Deputy Legal Advisor to the Centers
    for Disease Control and Prevention
    and the Agency for Toxic Sub-
    stances and Disease Registry,
    Atlanta, Georgia

J. VIRGIL PEAVY, M.S.
Senior Training Consultant, Public
    Health Practice Program Office,
    Centers for Disease Control
    and Prevention, Atlanta,
    Georgia

JACQUELYN A. POLDER, B.S.N., M.P.H.
Program Coordinator, Child Care
    Health and Safety Program, Centers
    for Disease Control and Prevention,
    Atlanta, Georgia

JEFFREY J. SACKS, M.D., M.P.H.
Medical Epidemiologist, Division of
    Unintentional Injury Prevention,
    National Center for Injury Preven-
    tion and Control, Centers for
    Disease Control and Prevention,
    Atlanta, Georgia

STEPHEN B. THACKER, M.D., M.Sc.
Director, Epidemiology Program
    Office, Centers for Disease
    Control and Prevention, Atlanta,
    Georgia

CARL W. TYLER, JR., M.D.
Assistant Director, Public Health
    Practice Program Office, Centers
    for Disease Control and Prevention,
    Atlanta, Georgia

STEPHANIE ZAZA, M.D.
Medical Epidemiologist, Epidemiol-
    ogy Program Office, Centers for
    Disease Control and Prevention,
    Atlanta, Georgia

I

BACKGROUND

1

FIELD EPIDEMIOLOGY DEFINED

Richard A. Goodman

James W. Buehler

First and foremost, the term "field epidemiology" must be defined. Other books[1-5] have addressed some of the practical and operational aspects of applying epidemiology in the field setting, but have not defined the discipline of field epidemiology. Therefore, the purpose of this chapter is to provide both a definition of this term and a framework for the concept of field epidemiology as it is used throughout this book.

The constellation of problems faced by epidemiologists who are called upon to investigate urgent public health problems gives shape to the definition of field epidemiology. Consider, for example, the following scenario: At 8:30 a.m. on Monday, August 2, 1976, Dr. Robert B. Craven, an Epidemic Intelligence Service officer assigned to CDC's Viral Diseases Division, received a telephone call from a nurse at a veterans' hospital in Philadelphia, Pennsylvania. The nurse had called to report two cases of severe respiratory illness (including one death) in persons who had attended the American Legion Convention in Philadelphia between July 21 and 24. Subsequent conversations with local and state public health officials revealed that, from July 26 to August 2, a total of 18 conventioneers had died, primarily from pneumonia. By the evening of August 2, an additional 71 cases had been identified among legionnaires. As a consequence of this information, a massive epidemiologic investigation was immediately initiated that involved public health agencies at the local, state, and federal levels. This problem became known as the first identified outbreak of legionnaires' disease and investigation of the problem led directly to the discovery of the gram-negative pathogen *Legionella pneumophila*.[6]

The legionnaires' disease outbreak and the public health response it triggered illustrate the raison d'être of field epidemiology. With this example in mind, we can define field epidemiology as the application of epidemiology under the following set of general conditions:

- The problem is unexpected.
- An immediate response may be demanded.
- Public health epidemiologists must travel to and work in the field to solve the problem.
- The extent of the investigation is likely to be limited because of the imperative for timely intervention.

While field investigations of acute problems share many characteristics with prospectively planned epidemiologic studies, they may differ in at least three important respects. First, because field investigations often start without clear hypotheses, they may require the use of descriptive studies to generate hypotheses before analytic studies are conducted to test these hypotheses. Second, as noted above, when acute problems occur, there is an immediate need to protect the community's health and address its concerns. These responsibilities drive the epidemiologic field investigation beyond the confines of data collection and analysis and into the realm of public health action. Finally, field epidemiology requires us to consider when the data are sufficient to take action rather than to ask what additional questions might be answered by the data.

The concepts and methods used in field investigations derive from clinical medicine, epidemiology, laboratory science, decision theory, skill in communications, and common sense. In this book, the guidelines and approaches for conducting epidemiologic field investigations reflect the urgency of discovering causative factors, the use of multifaceted methods, and the need to make practical recommendations.

UNIQUE CHALLENGES TO EPIDEMIOLOGISTS IN FIELD INVESTIGATIONS

An epidemiologist investigating acute problems in the field is faced by unique challenges that sometimes constrain the ideal use of scientific methods. In contrast to prospectively planned studies, which are based on carefully developed and refined protocols, field investigations must rely on data sources that are less readily controlled and that may literally change with each successive hour or day. In addition to potential limitations in data sources, other factors that pose challenges for epidemiologists during field investigations include sampling considerations, the availability of specimens, the impact of publicity, the reluctance of subjects to participate, and the conflicting pressures to intervene.

Data Sources

Field investigations often use information abstracted from a variety of sources, such as hospital, outpatient medical, or school health records. These records vary dramatically in completeness and accuracy among patients, health care providers, and facilities, since entries are made for purposes other than conducting epidemiologic studies. Thus, the quality of such records as sources of data for epidemiologic investigations may be substantially less than that of information obtained, for example, from standard, pretested questionnaires.

Small Numbers

In a planned prospective study, the epidemiologist determines appropriate sample sizes based on statistical requirements for power. In contrast, outbreaks can involve a relatively small number of persons, thereby imposing substantial restrictions on study design, statistical power, and other aspects of analysis. These restrictions, in turn, place limitations on the inferences and conclusions that can be drawn from a field investigation.

Specimen Collection

Because the field investigator usually arrives on the scene "after the fact," collection of necessary environmental or biological specimens is not always possible. For example, suspect food items may have been entirely consumed or discarded, a suspect water system may have been flushed, or ill persons may have recovered, thereby precluding collection of acute specimens. Under these conditions, the epidemiologist depends on the diligence of health care providers who first see the affected persons and on the recall of affected persons, their relatives, or other members of the affected community.

Publicity

Acute disease outbreaks often generate considerable local attention and publicity. In this regard, press coverage can assist the investigation by helping to develop information and identify cases or by promoting and helping to implement control measures. On the other hand, such publicity may lead affected persons and others in the community to form preconceptions about the source or cause of an outbreak, which, in turn, lead to potential biases in comparative studies or failure to fully explore alternate hypotheses. Parenthetically, media representatives in pursuit of the most current information on the investigation may demand a considerable amount of time—to the detriment of the field investigation itself.

Reluctance to Participate

While health departments are empowered to conduct investigations and gain access to records, voluntary and willing participation of involved parties is more conducive to successful investigations than is forced participation. In addition, persons whose livelihoods or related interests are at risk may be reluctant to cooperate voluntarily. This may often be the case for common-source outbreaks associated with restaurants and other public establishments, in environmental or occupational hazard investigations, or for health care providers suspected of being sources for transmission of infectious diseases such as hepatitis B. When involved parties do not willingly assist, delays may compromise access to and quality of information (e.g., by introducing bias and decreasing statistical power).

Conflicting Pressures to Intervene

Epidemiologists conducting field investigations must weigh the need for further investigation against the need for immediate intervention. However, the strong and varying opinions of affected persons and others in the community can interfere with the optimal scientific approach.

Two situations that may occur during an investigation merit comment, although they are not truly unique challenges to the field epidemiologist. First, on occasion, what appears to be a small, geographically well-defined epidemic turns out to be much larger in scope. This has been particularly true with salmonellosis epidemics that initially seem localized, only to be recognized regionally or nationally after reports appear in the media. Second, field investigations occasionally will turn up no evidence of an epidemic. Despite initial local concern, cries of epidemic, and a reasonable request by the local health officials, the field team may find no health problem at all.

REASONS AND STANDARDS FOR EPIDEMIOLOGIC FIELD INVESTIGATIONS

There are several reasons for doing field investigations:

- To control and prevent further disease
- To provide agreed-upon or statutorily mandated services
- To derive more information about interactions between the human host, the agent, and the environment
- To strengthen surveillance at the local level by assessment of its quality and by direct and personal contact, or to determine the need to establish a new surveillance system
- To provide training opportunities in field epidemiology

In judging an epidemiologic field investigation, paramount consideration should be given to the quality of the science. This should not be the sole standard, however, for the full range of limitations, pressures, and responsibilities imposed on the investigator must also be taken into account. The goal should be to maximize the scientific quality of the field investigation in the face of these limitations and competing interests.

The epidemiologist in the public sector must reconcile the multiple competing and/or conflicting interests and develop the most scientifically optimal study design possible under the circumstances. Sound judgment combined with a rigorous scientific effort will lead to a field investigation that meets the public's needs and also provides scientific data of the highest quality. Thus, the standards for an epidemiologic field investigation are that it (1) addresses an important public health problem in the community, as defined by standard public health measures (e.g., attack rates, serious morbidity, mortality) or community concern; (2) is timely; (3) examines resource needs early enough in the investigation and commits an appropriate level of public resources; (4) employs appropriate methods of descriptive and/or analytical epidemiology; (5) probes causality to the degree sufficient to enable identification of the source and/or etiology of the problem; and (6) establishes immediate control and long-term interventions.

REFERENCES

1. Last, J. M. (ed.) (1988). *Dictionary of epidemiology* (2nd ed.). Oxford University Press, New York.
2. Gregg, M. B., and Parsonnet, J. (1991). The principles of an epidemic field investigation. In *Oxford textbook of public health* (eds. W. W. Holland, R. Detels, G. Knox), vol. 4, pp. 399–415. Oxford University Press, New York.
3. Galbraith, N. S. (1985). The application of epidemiological methods in the investigation and control of an acute episode of infection. In *Oxford textbook of public health* (eds. W. W. Holland, R. Detels, G. Knox), vol. 4, pp. 3–21. Oxford University Press, New York.

4. Dixon, R. E. (1979). Investigation of endemic and epidemic nosocomial infections. In *Hospital infections* (eds. P. S. Brachman, J. V. Bennett), pp. 73–93. Little, Brown and Company, Boston.
5. Kelsey, J. S., Thompson, W. D., Evans, A. S. (1986). Epidemic investigation. In *Methods in observational epidemiology*, pp. 212–53. Oxford University Press, New York.
6. Fraser, D. W., Tsai, T. R., Orenstein, W., et al. (1977). Legionnaires' disease: Description of an epidemic of pneumonia. *New England Journal of Medicine*, 297, 1189–97.

2

A BRIEF REVIEW OF
BASIC PRINCIPLES OF EPIDEMIOLOGY

Carl W. Tyler, Jr.

"Epidemiology" has been defined as "The study of the distribution and determinants of health-related states or events in specified populations, and the application of this study to the control of health problems."[1] The four essential elements in the practice of epidemiology are (1) a requirement for scientific study, reasoning, and logic; (2) a focus on human populations; (3) a scope that encompasses all health issues, not just diseases or conditions for which biological inferences can be drawn; and (4) a concentration on control and prevention of health problems—the consequences of which, in the context of field epidemiology, will demand a set of actions. As the fundamental science of public health, epidemiology is not simply a field of study: it is a discipline in which the practitioner counts people or events, determines rates, and compares these rates in order to identify causes or risk factors that can be controlled or eliminated through public health intervention.

HISTORY

A few brief historical examples may give some idea of the scope of epidemiology. Around 300 B.C., Hippocrates emphasized the importance of the environment as a source of disease agents. In the 1600s, Graunt assembled 100 years' worth of

9

vital statistics into tables that defined the basic facts of human mortality. Louis changed medical practice in France in the 18th century by demonstrating the lack of therapeutic effect from bloodletting. In the mid-1800s, Holmes and Semmelweis described the transmission of puerperal sepsis both in the United States and Europe. In the 1850s, Snow helped reduce death from cholera in London by defining its waterborne transmission. Early in this century, Goldberger demonstrated the dietary etiology of pellagra. Doll and Hill established the causal link between cigarette smoking and lung cancer in a series of studies performed in England during the 1950s.

So the domain of epidemiology has expanded over time, and, quite literally, can now be defined only by one's concept of health. The World Health Organization defines health as not simply the absence of disease and debility but the presence of physical, mental, and social well-being. Acceptance of this definition requires epidemiologists to take responsibility not only for the infections of historic importance—such as plague, yellow fever, and epidemic typhus—but also for a number of new problems, for example, infections, such as Legionnaires' disease and AIDS; toxic agents, such as lead; chemical carcinogens, like the nitrosamines; natural disasters, such as floods and tornadoes; behavioral risk factors, such as cigarette smoking and alcohol misuse; violent behavior, such as homicide and suicide; and social problems, such as unplanned pregnancy among teenagers.

PURPOSES

In the broadest sense, epidemiology aims to increase our understanding of health and disease for the purposes of improving the former and controlling or preventing the latter. More specifically, however, epidemiologic methods are used to define the health of a community, to evaluate intervention methods, to determine individual risks and chances of morbidity and mortality, and to improve our understanding of clinical syndromes.

In the context of field epidemiology, epidemiologic methods are most often used to identify the agent(s) causing disease, modes of transmission, factors of susceptibility/risk/exposure, and environmental determinants. For example, in the epidemic of legionnaires' disease in Philadelphia in 1976, epidemiologists deduced from their studies that the causative agent resided in the air-conditioning system of the Bellevue-Stratford Hotel; that the agent was transmitted via the airborne route; that being a legionnaire put one at increased risk of disease; and that, in the majority of cases, spending an hour or more in the hotel's lobby was the necessary exposure for developing the disease. All of this was known 6 months before the agent was finally identified in a specimen of lung tissue from a fatal case of legionnaires' disease.[2] Similarly, epidemiology enabled public health epidemiologists to determine transmission mechanisms and groups at increased risk for acquired immunodeficiency syndrome (AIDS) and to develop recommendations for its prevention 3 years before the causative virus was identified.

CONCEPTS OF DISEASE OCCURRENCE

The Epidemiologic Triad

Developing a concept of how health problems occur is not easy. Some epidemiologists do it implicitly, keeping only mental notes. Others write it out. Nonetheless, the development of this concept or model is essential because it underlies the investigation of every health problem. Futhermore, it makes sense. Every health problem affects people, arises from a certain cause or causes, and occurs in a definite place. And whether disease or health problems occur depends upon a critical biological balance between all three elements.

These factors, then, make up what has been called the epidemiologic triad—the most fundamental model for conceptualizing health events used by epidemiologists (Figure 2–1).

The epidemiologic triad (agent, host, environment)

This triad is not only conceptually important but it has practical, everyday application in the real world of field investigations as well. To gain the necessary information to understand the problem in the field, the epidemiologist must have a thorough understanding of the characteristics of the host, the agent, and the en-

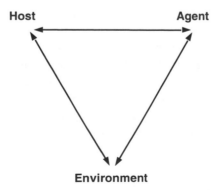

Figure 2–1. The epidemiologic triad (agent, host, and environment).

vironment in question. Such traits as age, gender, race, and occupation often provide the field epidemiologist with insight as to who is at risk and what may be the essential exposure. Likewise, an understanding of the agent's biological, physical, or chemical properties helps focus attention on some of the most likely explanations. However, when the agent is not known, a vital part of the triad is missing, making inferences much harder. Yet a thorough knowledge of the clinical and laboratory evidence can help fill this void. Last, all field investigations demand a comprehensive understanding of where things happened—environmental determinants such as the physical, biological, social, and economic factors that may have allowed or promoted interaction between host and agent.

Modes of Transmission

Epidemiology, as applied during the investigation of an outbreak of infectious disease, directs its attention toward defining the nature of the agent or agents, the source of same, the mode of transmission, and who is at risk and what exposure produced the disease.

For communicable diseases, knowing the portal of exit of an agent from its reservoir or source, the mechanism of its transmission, and its portal of entry into a susceptible host often give information critical for prevention and control. There are two basic modes by which agents may affect a susceptible host—direct and indirect. With infectious diseases, direct transmission occurs with immediate and direct transfer of an agent to a host by an infected person or animal. Touching, kissing, biting, or sexual intercourse are classic examples of direct transmission. Transfer of large airborne droplets of contaminated secretions is also considered a direct means of transmission, because the droplets travel only a few feet before contact. In a noninfectious disease setting, the host may have direct contact with the agent in the environment, as do children who ingest lead paint.

Indirect transmission may occur by three different mechanisms. Vehicle-borne transmission occurs through contaminated inanimate objects such as toys, bedding, cooking utensils, surgical instruments, food, water, or biological products like blood, tissues, or organs. Vector-borne transmission occurs through simple contamination by animal or arthropod vectors or their actual penetration of the skin or mucous membranes. Airborne transmission occurs when microbial, particulate, or chemical agents are aerosolized and remain suspended in air for long periods of time.

Epidemiologic Methods

Despite the increasingly complex nature of epidemiologic studies over the past 20 to 30 years, the basic methods used by both field and more academically oriented epidemiologists are the same, namely, description, hypothesis generation, and analysis.

Description

Virtually all epidemiologic studies entail observation of a population, counting health events, and describing them in the perspective of time, place, and person. This is often referred to as *descriptive epidemiology*.

Hypothesis generation

Once the "scenario" or the setting of the health event or epidemic is known, one can relate these findings to the population from which they came and ask the question: What do these data suggest or tell us? What analyses would help us answer these hypotheses?

Analysis

Often called *analytic epidemiology*, this stage of investigation includes determining rates of disease or exposure (performing long division), comparing these rates, and drawing inferences.

These studies center on human populations large and small and are characterized and analyzed by two basic approaches: the case control and the cohort methods of analyses.

Since field epidemiologists usually arrive in the field *after* the fact—namely, after a health event has occurred—their studies are usually *retrospective* in nature. They usually count and describe ill persons, develop hypotheses that, they hope, explain why illness occurred, and compare the ill (cases) with well people (controls). This is called a *case-control study*, and the analyses compare rates of exposure among the ill and the well persons. However, on occasion the field team may be called on to study a population *before* the health event has occurred, that is, *prospectively*. Here, the epidemiologists pose a hypothesis that a certain exposure causes a specific disease. Then exposed and nonexposed persons are studied to see if illness develops. This is called a *cohort study*, and the analyses compare rates of disease among the two study groups. (See Chapter 7 for detailed discussions of these kinds of studies.)

Another epidemiologic method sometimes used by field epidemiologists is the *cross-sectional* or *prevalence* study, when one may want to determine the prevalence of disease and exposures in a population at a moment in time. Although not giving information as to which event came first, such surveys can often help generate testable hypotheses (see Chapter 11).

Simple though these concepts and methods may appear, we shall see in later chapters that they can become complicated because the following simple questions do not always have straightforward answers. What is a case? Who is at risk?

What constitutes exposure? What is an appropriate comparison (control) group? What analytic methods should be used? And, inevitably, what do the analyses mean?

The Tasks of the Field Epidemiologist

The field epidemiologist has several responsibilities which, as a group, comprise a unique set of tasks.[3] These include surveillance, investigation, analysis, evaluation, and communication.

Surveillance

In its simplest terms, surveillance is the detection of health problems through the appropriate collection of data, followed by its collation, analysis, interpretation, and dissemination. Surveillance is the first task of the field epidemiologist because it provides an ongoing means for detecting important health problems (see Chapter 3).

Investigation

Epidemic investigation is often triggered by effective epidemiologic surveillance at various levels of reporting. Other sources of key information may include, for example, the media, hospitals, or private practice. The basic steps of a typical field investigation are discussed in Chapter 6.

Analysis

Analyses of data in the field include choosing the appropriate method, reviewing descriptive information, determining and comparing rates, and drawing conclusions—all of which are discussed in detail in several chapters that follow.

Evaluation

Although not discussed specifically in this book, evaluation is an essential part of the practice of field epidemiology. Both case control and cohort methods of analyses are used in the field to evaluate prevention and control efforts such as vaccine efficacy and malaria control.

Other essential tasks

Finally, effective communication, human relations, and management skills are essential to any successful field investigation; all of these are dealt with in subsequent chapters of his book.

REFERENCES

1. Last, J. M. (ed.) (1988). *Dictionary of epidemiology* (2nd ed.), p. 42. Oxford University Press, New York.
2. Fraser, D. W., Tsai, T. R., Orenstein, W., et al. (1977). Legionnaires' disease: Description of an epidemic of pneumonia. *New England Journal of Medicine*, 297, 1189–97.
3. Tyler, C. W., Jr., Last, J. M. (1992). Epidemiology. In *Maxcy-Rosenau-Last Public health & preventive medicine* (13th ed.) (eds. J. M. Last, R. B. Wallace), p. 11. Appleton & Lange, Norwalk, Connecticut/San Mateo, California.

3

SURVEILLANCE

Stephen B. Thacker

The two previous chapters have reviewed the basic principles and practices of epidemiology and their use in a newly defined application of epidemiologic study, namely, field epidemiology. With or without the urgency to investigate, to make recommendations, or to take specific action, however, all epidemiologic studies obtain data on a study population and capture facts to analyze.

But for the public health epidemiologist and, in particular, the field investigator, getting timely health-related data, either in a hurry or an ongoing basis, carries a distinct implication—the idea of using information for action. The acquisition of such information for use in public health has been called *surveillance*.

Definition

There is no standard, universally accepted definition of "surveillance" in public health practice. However, the following definition is widely accepted:

> Public health surveillance (sometimes called epidemiologic surveillance) is the ongoing and systematic collection, analysis, and interpretation of outcome-specific data essential to the planning, implementation, and evaluation of public health practice, closely integrated with the timely dissemination of these data to those who need to know. The final link of the surveillance chain is the application of these data to the control and prevention of human disease and injury.

Some have likened the surveillance system to a nerve cell, which has an afferent arm that receives information, a cell body that analyzes the data, and an efferent arm that takes appropriate action. This analogy is particularly appropriate in the context of field investigations, where surveillance must very often be started quickly to get the necessary data so that the right action can be taken.[1,2]

Background

After the discoveries of infectious disease agents in the late 1800s, the first use of scientifically based surveillance concepts in public health practice was the monitoring of contacts of persons with serious communicable diseases—such as plague, smallpox, typhus, and yellow fever—to detect the first signs and symptoms of disease and to begin prompt isolation. For many decades this was the function of foreign quarantine stations not only of the U.S. Public Health Service but quarantine agencies throughout the world.

In the late 1940s, Alexander D. Langmuir, M.D., then the chief epidemiologist of the Communicable Disease Center—now the Centers for Disease Control and Prevention (CDC)—began to broaden the concept of surveillance. Although surveillance of persons at risk of specific disease continued at quarantine stations, Langmuir and his colleagues changed the focus of attention to diseases, such as malaria and smallpox, rather than individuals. They emphasized rapid collection and analysis of data on a particular disease, with quick dissemination of the findings to those who needed to know.[3]

Now this credo of rapid reporting, analysis, and action applies to nearly a hundred infectious diseases and health events of noninfectious etiology nationally. Many ongoing systems of reporting have originated from national emergencies such as contaminated lots of polio vaccine (the so-called Cutter incident of 1955), the Asian influenza epidemic of 1957, shellfish-associated hepatitis A in 1961, and toxic shock syndrome in 1980. Within days of the investigation of L-tryptophan–associated eosinophilia-myalgia syndrome (EMS) in 1990, a national reporting system was put into place.

Types of Surveillance

Surveillance has been classified historically as either active or passive. *Passive* (or provider-initiated) surveillance refers to data supplied to a health department based on a known set of rules or regulations. For example, state laws or regulations in the United States require that physicians report certain diseases (mostly communicable) to a local health department. In turn, these reports may be sent to state health departments and on to CDC or the Public Health Service. Most surveillance systems throughout the world are passive, because this type is cheaper and easier for the health department to operate. In general, however, passive systems seriously undercount the occurrence of most reportable diseases.

In *active* surveillance (or health department–initiated surveillance), which is also based on certain regulations, the health agency regularly solicits reports from various providers. Active surveillance is most commonly implemented in an epidemic setting like the 1976 epidemic of legionnaires' disease in Philadelphia or the more recent epidemic of EMS in the United States. A modification of these two types is an enhanced passive surveillance system, where active follow-up of each case is used to pursue other possible cases (i.e., contact tracing of sexually transmitted disease performed by investigators in local health departments). Clearly, then, the system of surveillance will vary by disease, source of report, and sense of urgency.

The various principles and practices relating to surveillance that are discussed in this chapter apply broadly to all surveillance efforts, but because of the time frame involved, some practices are more appropriate for field investigations— the primary focus of our attention. Others are more adaptable to what we refer to as "ongoing" or long-term surveillance systems, where there often is no real sense of urgency. Though there is a gray area between the two, the basic differences remain clear and logical.

PURPOSES OF SURVEILLANCE

Whether you are investigating an epidemic in the field or implementing a statewide program of prevention, surveillance is the cornerstone, the management tool, for public health practice. Like good business practice, good surveillance provides the data needed to give:

- An accurate assessment of the status of health in a given population
- A quantitative base to define objectives for action
- Measures to define specific priorities
- Data to define strategies
- Measures to evaluate interventions, programs, and outcomes
- Information to plan and conduct research

In short, surveillance data provide a scientific, factual basis for appropriate policy decisions in public health practice and allocation of resources.

DATA SOURCES

Before discussing how to start a surveillance system, let us look at some of the kinds of data that are often readily available in the field and where they can be found. The nature of the problem will determine which data are most appropriate to collect. If certain information is not available, you may have to get it yourself by using surveys or questionnaires (see Chapter 11). In either case, a simple, standardized method should be developed at the beginning, with the understanding that as the health problem becomes more clearly defined or circumstances change during the investigation, the surveillance system may need to be modified accordingly.

Mortality Data

Mortality data are regularly available at the local and state levels, and because of burial laws, mortality statistics can be used at the local level within a matter of days. Mortality data are available on a weekly basis from 121 large U.S. cities as part of a national influenza surveillance system. Maintained and published weekly by CDC in collaboration with local health jurisdictions, these mortality statistics come from cities that represent about 27 percent of the nation's population and give a useful, timely index of the extent and impact of influenza at local, state, and national levels.

Medical examiners and coroners are excellent sources of data on sudden or unexpected deaths. Data are available at the state or county level and include detailed information about the cause and nature of death that is unavailable on the death certificate. These data are especially valuable for surveillance of intentional and unintentional injuries as well as sudden deaths of unknown cause.

Another source is the National Mortality Followback Survey conducted periodically by the National Center for Health Statistics (NCHS) of CDC on a sample of knowledgeable informants to ascertain social and health information on decedents.

The quality of death certificate data may vary a great deal from location to location, state to state, and particularly country to country. Physicians' assessments of cause or causes of death are notoriously divergent at times, and even definitions of death, time of death, and words like "infant" are subject to considerable variation. So comparisons of mortality statistics between time frames and across geopolitical boundaries should be made with extreme caution and only after in-depth knowledge of local customs, changes in coding of death certificates, and advances in medical knowledge—to name some important considerations—has been obtained.

Morbidity Data

As with mortality statistics, most countries require reporting of certain diseases (usually infectious) considered important. In the United States, laws and regulations of each state health department list from 50 to 130 notifiable diseases (or conditions) that are reportable health events.[4] These data are used routinely and published for surveillance purposes at local, state, and national levels. Virtually all surveillance systems rely on physicians or health care providers for these reports. Unfortunately, most infectious diseases are underreported, and in the United States there is great variation in the sensitivity and specificity of infectious disease reporting among the 50 states. Priorities, available resources, and diseases peculiar to the region usually dictate the quality of morbidity data collected.

Of course, unrecognized, undiagnosed illness never enters the reporting loop. However, the sensitivity and specificity of reports of both infectious and noninfectious conditions tends to increase the more severe and more rare the disease. Reporting of diseases under intensive surveillance, such as measles and AIDS in the United States, can reach 90 percent sensitivity, but such levels of reporting are uncommon.

There are other sources of morbidity data that can prove useful in both ongoing systems of surveillance and in field situations. Private physicians are contacted by a variety of survey groups. The National Ambulatory Medical Care Survey, conducted periodically by NCHS, includes a random sample of office-based physicians stratified by region. The National Drug and Therapeutic Index, conducted by a private company, IMS America, is a similar sample. From both of these, you can get diagnostic, specialty, therapeutic, and disposition data. The Ambulatory Sentinel Practice Network, initiated by the North American Primary Care Research Group, is an example of a voluntary office-based system that looks at particular health problems selected on a periodic basis.

Hospital data are another useful source of surveillance information. The National Hospital Discharge Survey, conducted by NCHS and private abstracting services such as the Commission of Professional and Health Activities and the McDonnell-Douglas Corporation, provides data abstracted from hospital records. Information from these sources typically includes diagnosis, length of stay, operative procedures, laboratory findings, and costs. The Birth Defects Monitoring Program of CDC uses abstracts from over a thousand hospitals to monitor the occurrence of congenital malformations. The National Nosocomial Infection Surveillance System is a voluntary system comprising hospitals that report data to CDC on hospital-acquired infections.

Laboratory Data

Whether serving the interests of a single hospital, a local or state health department, or a national or international health agency, the laboratory has given the field epidemiologist invaluable information, particularly in infectious disease outbreaks. Data on increases in microbial isolates, recognition of rare or unusual sero- or biotypes, or even simply an increase in demands for laboratory facilities provide essential information on the detection and investigation of epidemics caused by such agents as *Salmonella*, *Shigella*, *Escherichia coli*, and *Staphylo-*

coccus. Pivotal information used for control and prevention efforts has also come from ongoing surveillance of influenza and poliomyelitis isolates as well as laboratory studies of lead and other environmental hazards. With the rapid sophistication of laboratory tools in environmental health, the laboratory is playing an increasingly important role in field investigations of such toxicants as lead, mercury, pesticides, and volatile organic compounds.

Individual Case Investigation

Because some infectious diseases have high ratios of inapparent to apparent disease, a single case should be considered a sentinel health event and should be investigated immediately. A single case of paralytic poliomyelitis or aseptic meningitis represents one- to two-hundred other cases of mild to subclinical disease elsewhere in the community. One full-blown case of arthropod-borne encephalitis or dengue reflects tens, if not hundreds, of other cases as yet unrecognized or unreported. Recall, too, the variability of individual response to toxic exposures. A single clinical case of intoxication should alert you to the possibility of unrecognized exposures in the family or in the neighborhood. Similarly, a single case of some chemical or heavy metal poisoning, such as mercury-induced acrodynia, could be an indication of a potentially widespread risk.

Epidemic Reporting

Sometimes it is easier, more practical, and more useful to count epidemics rather than single cases of disease. This is particularly true of common diseases that have epidemic potential, that may be poorly reported, and, in some instances, diseases that have a wide clinical spectrum. Probably the best example is influenza. Indeed, one of the time-honored methods of tracking influenza includes several degrees of involvement assessed by each state. They will describe influenza levels as isolated cases, sporadic outbreaks, outbreaks affecting less than half of the counties in the state, and outbreaks affecting over half of the state's counties. Not rigorous science, but very useful. Rubella, rubeola, varicella, and dengue can be grossly assessed in this fashion—primarily to inform the public but also to indicate where to direct control or prevention efforts. In fact, during the smallpox eradication program of West Africa in the early 1970s, the field teams stopped counting cases; they counted only epidemics, defined as one or more cases. This saved much time and effort, focusing most of the resources on control.

Sentinel Systems

Existing systems of morbidity reporting should be sensitive and specific enough for you to detect early the appearance of an outbreak of an epidemic. For many reasons, however, not all such systems are that good. Also, some diseases of public health importance are not reportable conditions. No matter what the reason for inadequate reporting, there may be times when you should consider starting a sentinel system—a simple, relatively sensitive way of early detection and monitoring.

Again, probably the best example of this kind of surveillance has been influenza. Many states do not require physician reports of influenza, so that when epidemics are impending and it is considered important to know when they arrive, the state will ask or even pay selected physicians to report influenza cases on a daily basis. Usually, these kinds of voluntary systems are not statistically valid. Selection is usually based on willingness to cooperate and geographic location—both very practical and compelling reasons. In some countries, because diagnostic capabilities in remote areas barely exist, the sentinel system will merely require reports of "unusual events."

Knowledge of Vertebrate and Arthropod Vector Species

In many arboviral infections, for example, generally with high inapparent to apparent disease, humans represent an incidental or dead-end host and contribute insignificantly to transmission of the disease. Therefore, an important adjunct to or surrogate for human disease surveillance is the monitoring of nonhuman vertebrate hosts and species. In areas where human surveillance is poor or nonexistent, this may be the only reasonable way to document the introduction and spread of disease.

Similarly, illness in vertebrate or invertebrate animals may reflect exposure to environmental toxins before clinical disease appears in human populations. In circumstances where toxic exposures are thought to be increased, regular communication should be established between health officers, the veterinary community, and agencies responsible for monitoring other animal and insect populations.

Surveys of Health in General Populations and Special Databases

Although not frequently used in field investigation settings, several databases provide baseline or background incidence and prevalence information that may be helpful in the assessment of the magnitude of a problem under study. The National Health and Nutrition Examination Survey (NHANES) is a periodic survey conducted by CDC that includes clinical examination and laboratory data as well as demographic and medical history information. NHANES has been conducted three times since 1971. NHANES III began in 1988 and was completed in 1994. The National Health Interview Survey of NCHS is a continuing survey of nearly 50,000 civilian households that collects information on illness, disability, health service utilization, and activity restriction. The Behavioral Risk Factor

Surveillance System conducted by state health departments in collaboration with CDC is a telephone survey in approximately forty-five states that gathers information on tobacco use, alcohol use, seat belt use, hypertension, and weight. The National Ambulatory Medical Case Survey (NAMCS) is a national probability sample of visits to office-based physicians that began in 1974. The last survey was done in 1989 on 2,500 physicians, where data were collected on diagnosis, symptoms, drugs, and referrals.

There are several other national surveillance systems with distinctive features that may be considered before starting a surveillance system or performing a field study. The National Cancer Institute funds the Surveillance Epidemiology and End Results (SEER) system, a group of cancer registries in 11 geographic areas of the United States that collect information on cancer, histologic type, site, residence, and relevant demographic information. This information is particularly useful when one is called upon to investigate clusters of cancer in the field. The National Electronic Injury Surveillance System (NEISS) is a stratified random sample of hospital emergency rooms sponsored by the Consumer Products Safety Commission that collects continuous reports on product-related injuries and also carries out some special studies on problems such as injuries related to fire and motor vehicle accidents. The Fatal Accident Reporting System (FARS), initiated by the National Highway Traffic Safety Administration, collects information on fatal crashes occurring on public roadways. The National Accident Sampling System (NASS) is a random sample of police-reported traffic crashes in the United States. Finally, the Environmental Protection Agency compiles air monitoring data from 51 U.S. areas on six primary air pollutants to monitor compliance with the Clean Air Act. These various data sources have been used to combine health-event and risk-factor data for surveillance purposes.

Also be aware that medical school researchers, university hospitals, and voluntary organizations such as the Cystic Fibrosis Foundation collect and maintain incidence and prevalence data on a variety of health conditions that could be sources of valuable information during an investigation in the field.

Demographic and Environmental Factors

As in all epidemiologic investigations, you must know the basic demographic characteristics of the population at risk (i.e., number, age, gender distribution), among the many important variables. Without these data, no rates can be determined. That is to say, you must have a denominator to calculate rates of illness or exposure. In some instances, these data are not readily available, and they must be obtained during the field investigation. However time-consuming and expensive they may be to acquire, demographic data are indispensable; without them, valid comparisons of populations and exposures are impossible.

You may also need to document such characteristics as heat, cold, airflow, humidity, rainfall, and other environmental determinants that predispose to disease or injury during your investigations.

LEGAL ISSUES

Before establishing any surveillance system, be it an emergency system during a field investigation or a process of continued monitoring for months or years to come, you should first be very clear about the legal aspects of such a plan (see Chapter 14). In most instances, surveillance is conducted under the aegis of state health laws or regulations, so be careful to avoid any activities that violate such statutes. In epidemic investigations, the field team is usually given oral approval for setting up emergency surveillance systems; but when long-term programs of surveillance are being considered, you may have to obtain written clearance from the appropriate authorities.

Issues such as confidentiality and the public's right to know can be in conflict with each other, and these must be carefully considered at all steps in the surveillance process. Similarly, you must recognize who will be affected at each level of surveillance, including individuals in the community; patients (both inside and outside of institutions); practitioners, including physicians, nurses, and others involved in the health care delivery system; members of the local health department; and, of course, members of one's immediate staff. Failure to recognize potential conflicts of interest or lack of acceptability to any of these persons could derail the surveillance process.

HOW TO ESTABLISH A SURVEILLANCE SYSTEM

Goals

At the beginning, you need to understand clearly the purpose of establishing or maintaining a surveillance program. You should know which surveillance data are necessary and how and when they are to be used. A particular surveillance program may have more than one goal, including monitoring the occurrence of fatal and nonfatal disease, evaluating the effect of a public health program, or detecting epidemics for control and prevention activities. These needs, then, may require multiple surveillance systems to monitor a single condition, such as data to track morbidity, mortality, laboratory tests, exposures, risk factors, and so on. No matter what the goal, you must ask these questions: What action will be taken? What will be done with the data and the analyses? Without specific answers to these questions to guide the development of the surveillance system, the data collected may not be relevant or adequate. There must be a specific, action-oriented commitment, otherwise there is no point in bothering.

Personnel

It is essential to know not only who is responsible for overseeing the surveillance activities but also who will be providing the data, collecting and tabulating the data, analyzing and preparing the data for display, and, finally, who will be interpreting these data and disseminating them to those who need to know. In the field, you will likely know personally who these people are. In longer-range systems, which you will be implementing or orchestrating at some distance, these key people will probably be names only.

The entire surveillance system in a small area may have only one person doing essentially all these tasks. At the state, regional, and national levels, several persons will likely be involved in the surveillance of specific health events. In the setting of an acute outbreak, a large number of people at various professional levels may be involved in starting and conducting the necessary active surveillance. As time progresses and the epidemic becomes better understood, the participants will likely assume a better-defined role.

Case Definition

Use as clear and as simple a case definition as possible.[5] Ideally, it should be practical and should include quantifiable criteria. Minimal criteria for the definition of a case must be made explicit. The essential clinical and laboratory information that is desirable for surveillance purposes should be stated. During the course of an epidemic investigation, the case definition is often broad, sometimes depending on clinical and epidemiologic criteria in the absence of laboratory data. As the grasp of the disease process improves, a more refined definition may be used. In this context, distinguish confirmed cases from probable or possible cases, for, with the proper analysis, this often enhances an understanding of the causes of an outbreak while not losing sight of its scope and impact.

The Human Element in Surveillance

After you have designed and developed the surveillance system and are prepared to start, think of the human element involved. The system should be acceptable to all who play a part in the collection, analysis, dissemination, and use of the data. Be sure to make some personal contact—not only with those who supply the data but also with those who collect and analyze them. Successful systems have almost always included personal contact as an essential ingredient. An occasional visit, particularly to those providing the data, enhances interest and a sense of purpose, provides faces and names to remember, "humanizes" an otherwise often impersonal activity, gives the participants visibility, recognizes their importance, makes people glad they belong, and, in short, builds and supports a team—an absolute essential in any field investigation. At the beginning, if possible, you should also make contact with potential users of surveillance data to incorporate their needs into the collection, analysis, and dissemination process. From a strict management viewpoint, this means planning for travel costs in your budget.

Get the System Started

A final element in establishing a surveillance system is the need to get the system going. During an epidemic, this need is obvious. When reports of toxic shock syndrome began to appear in unprecedented numbers in early 1980, it became clear that a surveillance system was essential to assess the magnitude of the epidemic as well as the nature and distribution of cases. The same was true, of course, with AIDS the following year and EMS 10 years later. In any setting, however, try to engender a sense of the health event's importance in order to stimulate and maintain interest in studying it.

In establishing a long-term or ongoing system, a natural tendency at the start will be to make the system as specific and sensitive as humanly possible. Logical and defensible though this attitude may be, do not let it stand in the way of getting the system off the ground. Many a system has languished for months, even years, because of needless worry over a missing or misclassified case or two, thus losing interest, cooperation, and potential impact. Get the system moving; get the team energized and committed. You can always refine the system as it progresses. Remember, surveillance is a fluid process—as populations or health problems change, the surveillance system must adapt. If you know this, you will overcome a real tendency to wait or postpone starting the system until everything is scientifically perfect. Finally, because surveillance needs always change, one should also establish some kind of ongoing mechanism to monitor and evaluate the surveillance process.

ANALYSIS AND DISSEMINATION OF SURVEILLANCE DATA

As with all descriptive epidemiologic data, surveillance information must be analyzed in terms of time, place, and person. Apply simple tabular and graphic techniques for display and analysis (see Chapter 6). More sophisticated methods such as cluster and time-series analyses and computer mapping techniques may be appropriate at some point in time, but concentrate initially on simple presentations.

Critical to the usefulness of surveillance systems is the timely dissemination of surveillance data to those who need to know. Whatever format is chosen, be sure to define the audience clearly. Its composition will affect data collection and interpretation as well as the dissemination process. Distribute the data in a regular and timely manner so that control and prevention measures can be implemented. Remember that some of "those who need to know" include policymakers and administrators—people with little epidemiologic knowledge or background. So make the reports simple and easy to understand. Finally, recognize in print those who have contributed to the surveillance. People like to see their names in print, and people like to belong—it helps justify their role in the prevention process. Recognizing people by name gives them not only credit but a degree of responsibility as well.

Dissemination of Findings during a Field Investigation

In the field setting, particularly in large epidemics or epidemics covering large geographic areas, it is often very useful to print a daily or semiweekly surveillance report. It informs all interested parties; it is useful to give to the media (thus minimizing interviews); it helps avoid misinformation and misunderstanding; it identifies the "players"; it gives credit to those who deserve it; it identifies who is responsible for what; and it serves as a very useful diary of what was done, why, and what was found. In short, such a surveillance report serves as an extremely important management tool. Again, however, keep it simple, emphasizing tables, charts, and figures, with minimal text. To some degree, let the report speak for itself.

Dissemination of Findings from Ongoing Surveillance Systems

Many countries publish and distribute weekly, biweekly, or monthly reports of information relating to public health. CDC gives information to those who need to know through the *Morbidity and Mortality Weekly Report* (*MMWR*) and through the *MMWR*'s surveillance summaries, Recommendations and Reports, and Annual Summary of Notifiable Diseases as well as special, condition-specific reports. State and local health departments often have their own reports, analogous to those of the *MMWR*, that are disseminated to health care providers and other interested persons in the relevant states or communities. Also, surveillance data are analyzed and published in the medical literature, although the timeliness of these papers may often leave a good deal to be desired.

USES OF SURVEILLANCE DATA

Although we have already discussed the general purposes of surveillance activities, it may be useful to outline some additional uses of such systems, particularly those that are long range.

Portrayal of Natural History of Disease

Surveillance data are often used to identify or verify perceived trends in health problems. For example, the reported occurrence of malaria in the United States over the past 50 years has shown the impact of improved diagnosis, importation of cases from foreign wars, and the impact of both increased international travel by U.S. citizens and foreign immigration (Figure 3–1).[6] At the local, and to a lesser degree national level, surveillance data are used to detect epidemics that lead to control and prevention activities.

Test Hypotheses

In the day-to-day monitoring of health problems in a community, you often cannot wait to do special studies. So whatever data are available must be analyzed. Although the information may not be ideal for analysis, it can often be used to test certain hypotheses. For example, the impact of school entry laws in the United States was anticipated to change the patterns of reported cases by age. Indeed, it was found that within 2 years, the peak incidence of measles changed from school-aged children (10 to 14 years of age) before widespread adoption of these laws in 1980, to children below age 5 (Figure 3–2).[7]

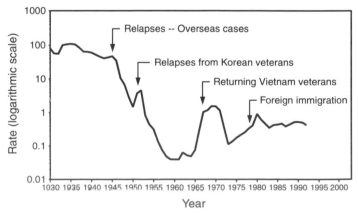

Figure 3–1.   Rate (reported cases per 100,000 population) of maleria–United States, 1930-1992. *Source:* CDC (1992).[6]

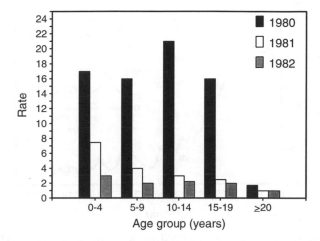

Figure 3-2. Estimated rate (cases per 100,000 population) of measles, by age group and year—United States, 1980-1982. *Source:* CDC (1983).[7]

Identify and Evaluate Control Measures

Surveillance data are used to quantify the impact of intervention programs. For example, they have demonstrated the decrease in poliomyelitis rates following the introduction of both the inactivated and oral polio vaccines (Figure 3–3)[8] and the effect of broad-based community interventions such as increased legal age of driving and seat belt laws.

Monitor Changes in Infectious Agents

In hospital and health department laboratories, various infectious agents are monitored for changes in bacterial resistance to antibiotics or antigenic composition. The detection of penicillinase-producing *Neisseria gonorrhoeae* in the United States has provided critical information for the proper treatment of gonorrhea (Figure 3–4).[9] The National Nosocomial Infection Surveillance System monitors the occurrence of hospital-acquired infections, including changes in antibiotic resistance. Another example has been the detection of the continual change in the structure of the influenza virus—information vital to vaccine formulation.

Monitor Isolation Activities

The traditional use of surveillance was to quarantine persons infected with or exposed to a particular disease and to monitor their health status. While this measure is rarely used today, isolation and surveillance of individuals is done for

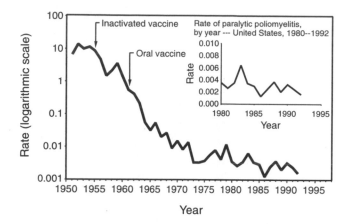

Figure 3–3.   Rate (reported cases per 100,000 population) of paralytic poliomyelitis—United States, 1951–1992. *Source:* CDC (1992).[6]

patients with multidrug-resistant tuberculosis and those suspected of having serious, imported diseases such as the hemorrhagic fevers.

Detect Changes in Health Practice

Surveillance has been used to monitor health practices such as hysterectomy, cesarean delivery, mammography, and tubal sterilization. The surveillance of such practices and health care technologies has been increasing in public health in recent years.[10]

Planning Activities

Surveillance data have served as the cornerstone of epidemiologic and public health practice. Representative and relevant data give information that helps design actions. This provides the necessary framework for the actual management of public health programs. For example, surveillance data have been kept on the location of Southeast Asian refugees in the United States in order to provide the appropriate public health services for the diagnosis and treatment of tuberculosis, a problem of particular concern to that population.

EVALUATION OF A SURVEILLANCE SYSTEM

It is not the purpose of this chapter to describe how to evaluate a surveillance program; its aim is only to present the basic essentials that need to be examined.

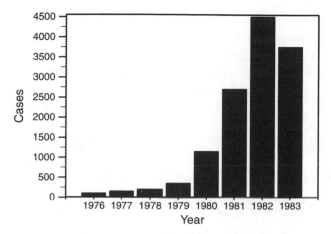

Figure 3-4. Cases of penicillinase-producing *Neisseria gonorrhoeae*–United States, 1976–1983. *Source:* CDC (1983).[9]

Surveillance systems should be evaluated at three levels: (1) public health importance of the health event; (2) usefulness and cost of the surveillance system; and (3) explicit attributes of the quality of the surveillance system, including sensitivity, specificity, representativeness, timeliness, simplicity, flexibility, and acceptability.

The decision to establish, maintain, or deemphasize a surveillance system should be guided by assessments based on these criteria. Ultimately, the decision rests on whether a health event under surveillance is a public health priority and whether the surveillance system is useful and cost-effective.[11]

SUMMARY

Public health surveillance is the cornerstone of public health practice, providing the scientific and factual database essential to informed decision making. Surveillance data have many uses; in general, however, they are needed to assess the health status of a population in order to set public health priorities and determine appropriate actions. Surveillance is based on morbidity, mortality, and risk-factor data, often from multiple sources.

Surveillance systems are established for the identification of specific outcomes, such as those resulting from a disease or injury, and must have clearly expressed goals. Explicit case definitions are at the core of a good surveillance system. The initiation and maintenance of any successful surveillance system will reflect recognition of the human element in surveillance practice—in data collection, analysis, and dissemination. Insensitivity to the people involved in such a system dooms it to failure.

In field investigations, where time may be a critical factor, surveillance data must be collected quickly, recognizing the need for simple, practical systems that will give scientifically valid data for immediate action.

Effective systems of public health surveillance are evaluated regularly on the basis of their usefulness in public health practice.

REFERENCES

1. Thacker, S. B., Choi, K., Brachman, P. S. (1983). The surveillance of infectious diseases. *Journal of the American Medical Association*, 249, 1181–85.
2. Thacker, S. B., Berkelman, R. L. (1988). Public health surveillance in the United States. *Epidemiologic Reviews*, 10, 164–90.
3. Langmuir, A. D. (1963). The surveillance of communicable diseases of national importance. *New England Journal of Medicine*, 268, 182–92.
4. Chorba, T. L., Berkelman, R. L., Safford, S. K., et al. (1989). Mandatory reporting of infectious diseases by clinicians. *Journal of the American Medical Association*, 262, 3018–26.
5. Wharton, M., Chorba, T. L., Vogt, R. L., et al. (1990). Case definitions for public health surveillance. *Morbidity and Mortality Weekly Report*, 39 (RR-13), 1–43.
6. Centers for Disease Control and Prevention (1992). Summary of notifiable diseases, United States, 1991. *Morbidity and Mortality Weekly Report*, 41, 38.
7. Centers for Disease Control (1983). Annual summary 1983: Reported morbidity and mortality in the United States. *Morbidity and Mortality Weekly Report*, 32, 33.
8. Centers for Disease Control and Prevention (1992). Summary of notifiable diseases, United States, 1992. *Morbidity and Mortality Weekly Report*, 41, 46.
9. Centers for Disease Control (1983). Annual summary 1983: Reported morbidity and mortality in the United States. *Morbidity and Mortality Weekly Report*, 32, 25.
10. Thacker, S. B., Berkelman, R. L. (1986). Surveillance of medical technologies. *Journal of Public Health Policy*, 7, 363–77.
11. Klaucke, D. N., Buehler, J. W., Thacker, S. B., et al. (1988). Guidelines for evaluating surveillance systems. *Morbidity and Mortality Weekly Report*, 37 (S-5).

II

THE FIELD INVESTIGATION

4

OPERATIONAL ASPECTS OF
EPIDEMIOLOGIC INVESTIGATIONS

Richard A. Goodman
Michael B. Gregg
Robert A. Gunn
Jeffrey J. Sacks

An epidemiologic field investigation entails considerably more effort than simply following the recommended steps outlined in Chapter 5. Besides the necessary collection, tabulation, and analyses of the data, numerous and at times overwhelming operational issues must be addressed as well. This chapter describes certain critical operational and management principles that apply before, during, and after the fieldwork. These include the evaluation of and response to an invitation to perform an investigation and the proper preparation—including collaboration and consultation; basic administrative instructions before departure to the field; and, finally, the initiation, implementation, and aftermath of the field investigation. These considerations extend far beyond the scientific work of the investigators. However, if they are not addressed, the field investigation can be done only with great difficulty or may even fail.[1]

THE INVITATION

An essential consideration is the need to have a formal request for assistance from an official who is authorized to request help. In the United States, the responsibility for public health rests primarily within the state and local health agencies. In most instances, the state epidemiologist has the authority and responsibility for major epidemiologic field investigations and decides whether to investigate independently or to seek help elsewhere. Other persons or authorities may also be involved in generating a request for epidemiologic assistance, including those in institutional hierarchies (e.g., nursing homes, hospitals, and businesses), as well as institutions with special jurisdiction, including prisons, military facilities, cruise ships, and reservations for Native Americans. For international problems, the determination of authority for a request may be considerably more complicated and may involve, for example, ministries of health, multinational organizations (e.g., the World Health Organization), and others (see Chapter 17).

The relationships between larger and smaller health jurisdictions vary not only from state to state (or province to province) within countries but also from country to country. In general, the larger health jurisdictions help serve the smaller in time of need. Yet the sensitivities between these two authorities are often delicate, particularly as they relate to perceived competence, local jurisdiction, and ultimate authority. The health officers of the jurisdiction providing assistance must decide—on the basis of prevailing local-state amenities and agreements as well as their best judgment—what is the most appropriate response.

At the time of the initial request for assistance, you should attempt to determine three factors. First, what is the purpose of the investigation? Is the health department simply requesting more help to perform or complete the investigation? Has the health department been unable to determine the nature or source of disease or the mode of spread? Perhaps the health department wants to share the responsibility of the investigation with a more seasoned and knowledgeable health authority so as to be relieved of political or scientific pressure. Occasionally, legal or ethical issues may have become prominent in the early investigation, and you should be aware of this possibility. Rarely, an epidemic may even be declared or announced by health authorities or citizens. Assistance is then requested in order to publicize perceived adverse health conditions, to awaken state or national health leaders, or even to secure funds.

Second, and clearly related to the above, there is a need to determine specifically what the investigation is expected to accomplish. The team may be asked to confirm the findings already collected, collect new or different data for local analysis, or perform an entirely new investigation, including analysis and recommendations. And third, you should confirm that the requestor is authorized to invite assistance. Occasionally field studies have been aborted simply because those requesting assistance either had no authority to do so or state or national teams were investigating without local permission.

THE RESPONSE AND THE RESPONSIBILITIES

There are several reasons why field investigations should be done, if not encouraged:

- To control and prevent further disease
- To provide agreed upon or statutorily mandated services
- To derive more information about interaction between the human host, the agent, and the environment
- To strengthen surveillance at the local level through assessment of its quality and by direct and personal contact or to determine the need to establish a new surveillance system
- To provide training opportunities in field epidemiology[2]

If a decision is made to provide field assistance, the following points must be discussed with the local health official:

- What resources [including personnel] will be available locally?
- What resources will be provided by the visiting team?
- Who will direct the day-to-day investigation?
- Who will provide overall supervision and ultimately be responsible for the investigation?
- How will the data be shared and who will be responsible for their analysis?
- Will a report of the findings be written, who will write it, to whom will it go, and who will be the senior author of a scientific paper should one be written?

These are extremely critical issues, some of which cannot be totally resolved before the investigative team arrives on the scene. However, they must be addressed, discussed openly, and agreed upon as soon as possible.

PREPARATION

Collaboration and Consultation

Many field investigations require the support of a competent laboratory. Even if local laboratories are capable of processing and identifying specimens, you should immediately, upon being informed of the proposed investigation, contact your counterparts within your state or provincial laboratories. These laboratory scientists should be asked to provide any needed guidance and laboratory assistance. Now is the time to obtain assurance of cooperation and commitment rather than during the field investigation or near the end, when specimens have already been collected. The laboratorians must not only schedule the processing of specimens but must be asked to recommend what kinds of specimens are to be collected and how they should be collected and processed (see Chapter 18). There also may be substantive basic or applied research questions that could be appropriately addressed and answered during the field investigation. Discuss these issues in detail with these professionals, and make every effort to enlist their interest and support.

Advice on statistical methods may also be sought at this time as well. The same consideration applies to contacting other health professionals, such as veterinarians, mammalogists, entomologists, and environmental experts whose expertise can be crucial to a successful field investigation. Moreover, give serious consideration to including such professionals on the investigative team. Determine whether they should be part of the initial team so that appropriate data and particularly specimens can be collected at the same time as other relevant epidemiologic information.

Information specialists can also be extremely important in the overall management of a field investigation (see Chapter 13). Because large outbreaks will likely attract moderate local or regional attention in the media, the presence of an experienced and knowledgeable information officer who can respond to public inquiries and meet the media on a regular basis can be invaluable. Consider including secretarial and/or administrative personnel on the investigating team—not only to use their services but to expose them to a real-life situation. They will return home with a better understanding of fieldwork and with an increased ability to support future field investigations.

Basic Administrative Instructions and Notification

Once the field team has been chosen, certain key measures should be taken.

- Identify the team leader and the person to whom he or she should report regularly at the "home base."
- Try to arrange in advance an initial meeting with the requester or with persons either designated or identified by the requester. This will ensure that local authorities are not surprised by an unexpected arrival. In addition, this step underscores for all parties the need for advance planning and orderliness in the investigation—in essence, it sets a tone for the conduct of the investigation.
- Before leaving for the field, a senior member of the team should write a memorandum. It should summarize how and when the request was made, what information was provided by the local health department, what is the agreed upon purpose of the investigation, what are the commitments of both health authorities, who is on the field team, and when the latter is expected to arrive in the field. This memorandum should be distributed to key personnel in both health offices and to others who need to know. This kind of communication should assure proper notification that is necessary to prevent redundant responses (i.e., to avoid "crossing wires"), as well as to

identify expertise and resources from other programs that may contribute to the investigation. Basic programmatic jurisdictions and interests must also be respected, and some programs and staff simply want or need to know as a courtesy. Even when a problem does not directly involve a state (for example, as in the case of a prison or a military facility), state and local officials are generally notified because of possible ramifications to populations in surrounding communities. For example, at CDC, internal notification is effected using a standard memorandum to notify the CDC director, other senior managers, the Office of Public Affairs, and other key programs. In addition, CDC ensures that an essential list of key public health officials in the state and local health department that has issued the request are informed about the invitation. Depending on the circumstances and scope of the problem, other federal agencies and even other states may be notified about the problem and pending investigation.

- Last, before departing for the field, all members of the investigative team should review a basic checklist to be sure they have materials and aids that are essential for field operations and have covered fundamental travel and logistic considerations. Such items include, for example, background journal articles, statistical references, portable microcomputers, cameras and film, dictaphones and tape, credit cards, and travel and lodging reservations.

INITIATION OF THE INVESTIGATION

A key concept for the field team to keep in mind is the importance of the "consultant/collaborator" role and what that implies for an individual or team invited to provide assistance in an investigation. In general, the guiding principle should be that you are there to provide help, not simply to "take charge." Equally important, try to balance the focus of your investigation with the competing priorities in the local jurisdiction. While the immediate problem is your sole concern, the health authorities in the local jurisdiction must continue to address a myriad of other priorities and ongoing problems. This dichotomy can be appreciated if you and your team try to take the local point of view early in the investigation.

Once on site, you should meet promptly with the authority who requested assistance—usually the state or local epidemiologist or a program director. Essential steps that must be taken at this initial meeting include the following:

- Review and update the status of the problem
- Identification/review of primary contacts
- Identification of a principal collaborator who can also serve as a "guardian angel" during the investigation

- Identification of local resources (e.g., office space, clerical support, assistance for surveys, and laboratory support)
- Creation of a method and schedule for providing updates to local authorities and headquarters
- A review of sensitivities, including potential problems with institutions and individuals (e.g., hospitals, administrators, practitioners, and local public health staff) likely to be encountered during the investigation (Ideally, you should take the day or so needed to meet the requesting authority initially—so that key "doors" will be opened—rather than to spend valuable time later in the investigation mending bridges.)

During the initial meeting, you should also identify the appropriate local person to speak for the entire investigative team, when necessary. In general, the visiting team should try to avoid direct contact with the news media and should always defer to local health officials (see Chapter 13). The field team is essentially working at the request and under the aegis of the local health authorities. Therefore, it is the local officials who not only know and appreciate the local situation but also are the appropriate persons to comment on the investigation. In the most practical sense, the less the media make contact with you and your team, the more you can do at your own pace and discretion.

The work required to organize an investigation through this stage (i.e., starting travel and convening the initial meeting) is relatively straightforward and uncomplicated. In contrast, however, at least three factors will likely complicate the start of your scientific investigation: the effects of a new setting (i.e., you are an outsider and unfamiliar with the environment), the often intense pressure to solve the problem immediately and end the outbreak, and the queries of the media and other demands for your time. Thus, in short order, circumstances may change from tranquility and orderliness to a situation of pressure and confusion. To overcome the myriad potential distractions, you must maintain the proper perspective by adhering to the basics: focus the mission to collect data systematically; verify the diagnosis; and then proceed through case identification, orientation of data, and development and testing of hypotheses (see Chapter 5). Therefore, at the conclusion of the initial meeting, you should try to visit patients to verify the diagnosis through interviewing and, if necessary, through physical examination and review of laboratory data.

MANAGEMENT

Because of the potential complexity of field investigations as well as the distracting circumstances under which they are typically conducted, you may want to take the following approaches to ensure the systematic and orderly progression of the investigation. First, maintain lists of necessary tasks; check off those actions that have been completed and update the list at least twice daily. Second, communicate frequently with coworkers, the requesting authority, and the person designated to be the media contact; a team meeting should be held each day at a regularly scheduled time. Third, never hesitate to request additional help if required by the circumstances. Fourth, to ensure that the investigation will be completed, avoid setting a departure date in advance or succumbing to the pressure of family members to return earlier.

Investigations of large and complex problems may be particularly challenging for field teams and require even more rigorous organization of field operations. The following framework, reflected by the mnemonic SLACK OFF, was developed in 1986 by one of the authors (J.S.) during a complicated and protracted epidemiologic field investigation of a cluster of unexplained cardiopulmonary arrests. The methods and techniques used during the investigation were encompassed by this acronym to help organize and manage the activities of a large field team that worked with multiple data sets.

S—Shells (i.e., Table Shells)

- Begin at the end. In other words, ask: What are the questions to answer? Think in terms of who is at risk and what was the exposure that led to disease.
- Create the table shells (2x2 tables) needed to answer your questions. These shells help define what data you need and how to get them.
- Collect sufficient data to subsequently classify or stratify levels of exposure and outcome. Think quantitatively—for example:
  - How much (food or water)
  - How long (outdoors, in a room)
  - How sick (died, hospitalized, ambulatory)
- Remember that you may need to consult a statistician before collecting data.

L—Log Decisions

Record your decisions as you make them—it will ensure consistency and will make the study reproducible. This is particularly important in regard to case definitions and why certain criteria were used.

A—Accuracy

Remember the need for quality control measures such as training and monitoring of data collectors and abstractors, conducting error checks and validating data independently, and evaluating nonrespondents and missing records.

C—Communication

As mentioned above, there are different but necessary approaches to both internal (i.e., with colleagues and field team members) and external (i.e., the press) communications.

K—KISS (Keep It Simple, Stupid)

- Try to reduce the problem to one 2x2 table.
- Resist collecting more data than are needed (e.g., excessive clinical details).

O—Ongoing Writing

- Write down what got you there to begin with (i.e., a background section).
- Write while the investigation is ongoing—months later, you will have forgotten what you did.
- Write the methods while you are defining them—a decision log helps.

F—Filing

- Maintain and retain an inventory of data files.
- Protect the confidentiality of subjects.

F—Friendship

- Because field investigations are difficult—associated with long hours and great stress—make a special effort to maintain morale.
- Provide encouragement, positive reinforcement, and appreciation to those who participate.

DEPARTURE

Upon concluding the on-site field investigation, you should organize a departure meeting to include the requester, other key officials, and members of the investigation team. In addition to formally helping conclude the on-site work, the departure meeting enables you to debrief the requester on findings of the investigation, review preliminary recommendations, provide acknowledgments, and express appreciation to local hosts and collaborators. You should obtain any additional names, titles, and addresses for follow-up letters and correspondence. When possible, leave on site a preliminary report, but be certain to make a commitment to provide a complete written report within an agreed upon, specified time period.

The departure meeting may also be the most appropriate occasion for planning follow-up activities with the local organization. Such activities include the needs for additional studies, evaluation of control measures, analysis and maintenance of data collected during the investigation, plans for final reports and manuscripts (including discussion of authorship), and determining who is responsible for each of these different follow-up activities.

REPORTS

Written summaries of the investigation include both preliminary and final reports. The preliminary report fulfills the immediate obligation to the requesting authority; it should include a summary of methods used to conduct the investigation, preliminary epidemiologic and laboratory findings, recommendations, a clear delineation of tasks and activities that must be completed, and appropriate "thank yous." In addition to the preliminary report, which optimally should be delivered to the requester within 1 to 2 weeks of completion of the investigation, you should prepare follow-up letters to other principals (e.g., local health officials, coinvestigators, etc.) to inform them and to reinforce long-term relations.

The final reports should be written as quickly as possible—before you are called out to another epidemiologic field investigation! The final report should include complete and final data. In addition to a written final report, you should consider other methods or forums for communicating the findings of the investigation. Options include formal seminars for oral presentation to obtain critical feedback, reports for public health bulletins intended for public health practitioners, comprehensive articles for peer-reviewed journals, and presentations at professional meetings.

REFERENCES

1. Vaughan, J. P., Morrow, R. D. (eds.) (1989). *Manual of epidemiology for district health management*. World Health Organization, Geneva.
2. Gregg, M. B., Parsonet, J. (1989). The principles of an epidemic field investigation. In *Textbook of public health*, vol. III (2nd ed.) (eds. R. Detels, W. Holland, G. Knox). Oxford University Press, London, England.

5

CONDUCTING A FIELD INVESTIGATION

Michael B. Gregg

This chapter attempts to explain how to perform an epidemiologic field investigation. It focuses on a presumed point-source (common-source) epidemic, recognized and reported by local health authorities to a state (or provincial) health department. This is a typical setting that highlights the tasks that need to be performed. Although the scenario is one of an acute infectious disease epidemic in a community, the epidemiologic and public health principles apply equally well to investigations of noninfectious diseases.

BACKGROUND CONSIDERATIONS

Overall Purposes and Methods

As previously mentioned, the purposes of epidemiology include determining the cause or causes of a disease, its source, its mode of transmission, who is at risk of developing the disease, and which exposure or exposures predispose to the disease. Fortunately, in many outbreak investigations, the clinical syndromes are easily identifiable; the agents can readily be isolated and characterized; and the source, mode of transmission, and risk factors of the disease are usually well known and understood. Therefore, one is often quite well prepared for the field investigation. However, when the clinical diagnosis and/or laboratory findings are unclear, the task becomes much more difficult. This requires more careful consideration of the clinical presentation of disease in an effort to determine the source, mode of spread, and population or populations at risk. For example, bacterial contamination of food or water is usually manifest by signs and symptoms referable to the gastrointestinal tract. Pathogenic agents transmitted in air often affect the respiratory tract and sometimes the skin, eyes, or mucous membranes. Skin abrasions or lesions may suggest animal or insect transmission. Therefore the clinical manifestations of disease may serve as critical leads.

Regardless of how secure the clinical diagnosis may be, the investigator's thought process must include clinical, laboratory, and epidemiologic evidence. Together, these provide leads and pathways one may take or reject in order to discover the natural history of the epidemic.

Although you will perform several separate operations, in broad strokes the field epidemiologist really does two things. First, he or she collects information that describes the setting of the outbreak, namely: when people became sick, where they acquired disease, and what the characteristics of the ill people were. These are the descriptive aspects of the investigation. Often, simply by knowing these facts (and the diagnosis), one can determine the source and mode of spread of the agent and can identify those primarily at risk of developing disease. Common sense will often provide these answers, and relatively little, if any, further analysis is required.

On occasion, however, it will not be readily apparent where the agent resided, how it was transmitted, who was at risk of disease, and what the exposure was. Under these circumstances, a second operation, analytic epidemiology, must be used, which, one hopes, will provide the answers. Virtually all epidemiologic analyses require comparisons, usually of groups of persons—ill and well, exposed and not exposed (see Chapter 7). In epidemic situations, one usually compares ill and well people—both believed to have been at risk of disease—to determine what exposures ill people had that well people did not have. These comparisons are made by using appropriate statistical techniques (see Chapters 7 and 8). If the differences between ill and well persons are greater than one would expect by chance, one can draw certain inferences about why the epidemic occurred. In some situations, comparisons can be made between exposed persons and those not exposed to see if there are significant differences in rates of illness between the two groups.

The Pace and Commitment of a Field Investigation

An underlying theme throughout this chapter is the need to act quickly, establish clear operational priorities, and perform the investigation responsibly. This should not imply haphazard collection and inappropriate analysis of data but rather the use of simple and workable case definitions, case-finding methods, and analyses (see Chapter 4). Data collection, analysis, and the drafting of recommendations should be performed in the field. There is a strong tendency to collect what you think is the essential information in the field and then to retreat to "home base" for analysis—particularly with the availability of personal computers. Avoid this reflex at all costs. Such action will likely be viewed as lack of interest or concern or even as possessiveness by the local constituency. A premature departure also makes any further collection of data or direct contact with study populations and local health officials difficult or impossible. Once home, you lose the urgency and momentum to perform, the sense of relevancy of the epidemic, and, most of all, the totally committed time for the investigation. Every field investigation should be completed not only to the field team's satisfaction but particularly to the satisfaction of the local health department as well (see Chapter 9).

THE INVESTIGATION

Introduction

The ten basic tasks described here are presented in Table 5–1 in logical order. However, you may perform several of these functions simultaneously or in different order during the investigation. Control and prevention measures may even be recommended soon after beginning the investigation simply on the basis of intuitive reasoning and/or common sense. Sometimes the local officials know why the epidemic occurred, and you are there simply to supply a scientific basis for their conclusion. No two epidemiologists will take exactly the same pathway of investigation. Yet, in general, the data they collect, the analyses they apply, and the control and prevention measures they recommend will likely be similar.

Since our example of an epidemic is from a point source and may be nearly over before the field team arrives, the investigation in all likelihood will be retrospective. This should alert you to some fundamental aspects of any investigation that occurs "after the fact." First, because many illnesses and critical events have already occurred, virtually all information acquired and related to the epidemic will be based on memory. Health officers, physicians, and patients will likely have different recollections, views, or perceptions of what transpired. Information may conflict or may not be accurate, and it certainly cannot be expected to reflect the precise occurrence of past events. Like the clinician, the field epidemiologist may have to ask patients what they think made them sick and what they think caused the epidemic. Most critically, in parallel with medical practice, action may have to be taken without the benefit of all the desired data (see Chapter 9).

Table 5–1. The Ten Steps of a Field Investigation

---

1. Determine the existence of the epidemic.
2. Confirm the diagnosis.
3. Define a case and count cases.
4. Orient the data in terms of time, place, and person.
5. Determine who is at risk of becoming ill.
6. Develop a hypothesis explaining the specific exposure that caused disease and test this hypothesis by appropriate statistical methods.
7. Compare the hypothesis with the established facts.
8. Plan a more systematic study.
9. Prepare a written report.
10. Execute control and prevention measures.

For the young, inexperienced medical epidemiologist steeped in the tradition of molecule and millimole determinations, the "more-or-less" measurements of the field epidemiologist can initially be major hurdles to a successful field investigation. But however lacking in accuracy these data may be, they are often the only data available, and they must be collected, analyzed, and interpreted with care, imagination, and caution. Furthermore, you may not have seen the epidemiologic method work in real life. Unlike clinical medicine, where, in a matter of minutes to a few hours, the physical examination usually reinforces the history and the laboratory results usually reinforce both, there is often no immediate reinforcement of one's thought processes and activities in the field. It usually takes several days or a week before data start coming in that will reassure you that you are on the right track.

Determine the existence of an epidemic

Local health officials will usually know if more disease is occurring than would normally be expected. Since most local health departments have ongoing records that include comparisons by week, month, and year of communicable diseases and certain noninfectious conditions, one can easily determine if the observed numbers exceed the expected level. Although you may not have laboratory confirmation at this time, an increase in reported cases by local physicians is enough evidence to justify investigation. At this time, however, avoid the use of the terms "epidemic" or "outbreak," because these words are quite subjective. Local health officials take different views of the normal rise and fall in cases and whether changes in the pattern merit investigation.

You must be aware of artifactual causes of increases or decreases in reported cases, such as changes in local reporting practices, increased interest in certain diseases because of local or national awareness, a new physician or clinic in town, or changes in diagnostic methods. An excellent example of artifactual reporting occurred in southwest Florida in 1977 when a new physician in the community reported many cases of encephalitis in his practice. After extensive fieldwork by local, state, and federal epidemiologists, it became clear there was no epidemic but simply misdiagnoses by the physician.[1]

Sometimes, however, it may be difficult to document the existence of an epidemic. You may need to acquire absentee records from schools or factories or records of outpatient clinic visits and hospitalizations, laboratory records, or death certificates. A simple telephone survey of practicing physicians will strongly support the existence of an epidemic, as would a similar rapid survey of households in the community. In such quick assessments, you could ask about signs and symptoms rather than about specific diagnoses. Ask physicians or clinics if they are treating more people than usual with sore throats, gastroenteritis, fever with rash, for example, in order to obtain an index of disease incidence. Although not specific for any given disease, such surveys can often establish the existence of an epidemic. Sometimes it is extremely difficult to determine if there is an epidemic. Yet because of local pressures, the team may have to continue the investigation even if they believe no significant health problem exists.

Confirm the diagnosis

Confirm the clinical diagnosis by standard laboratory techniques such as serology and/or isolation and characterization of the agent. Do not try to use newly introduced, experimental, or otherwise not broadly recognized confirmatory tests—at least not at this stage in the investigation. If at all possible, visit the laboratory and verify the laboratory findings in person (e.g., talk to the technician, check the record books, and look at the gram stain yourself).

Not every reported case has to be confirmed in the laboratory. If most patients have signs and symptoms compatible with the working diagnosis and perhaps, 15 to 20 percent are laboratory-confirmed, you do not need more confirmation at this time. This is usually ample confirmatory evidence. See and examine several representative cases of the disease as well if at all possible. Clinical assumptions should not be made; the diagnosis should be verified by you or a qualified physician with you. Nothing convinces supervisors and health officers more than an eyewitness confirmation of clinical disease by you and the investigating team.

Define a case and count cases

Now try to create a workable case definition, decide how to find cases, and count them. The simplest and most objective criteria for a case definition are usually the best (e.g., fever, x-ray evidence of pneumonia, white blood cells in the spinal fluid, number of bowel movements per day, blood in the stool, or skin rash).

However, be guided by the accepted, usual presentation of the disease with or without standard laboratory confirmation in your case definition. Where time may be a critical factor in a rapidly unfolding field investigation, use a simple, easily applicable definition—recognizing that some cases will be missed and some noncases included. For example, in an epidemic of hepatitis A, a history of jaundice, fever, and an abnormal liver enzyme test should be quite adequate to start with. Later, you can refine the definition.

Some factors that can help to determine the levels of sensitivity and specificity of the case definition are the following:

- What is the usual apparent-to-inapparent clinical case ratio?
- What are the important and obvious pathognomonic or strongly clinically suggestive signs and symptoms of the disease?
- What microbiologic or chemical isolations, identification, and serologic techniques are easy, practical, and reliable?
- How accessible are the patients or those at risk? Can they be contacted again after the initial investigation for follow-up questions, examination, or serology?
- In the event that the investigation requires long-term follow-up, can the case definitions be applied easily and consistently by others not on the current investigating team?
- Is it absolutely necessary that all patients be identified during the initial investigation, or would only those seen by physicians or hospitalized suffice?

No matter what criteria are used, you must apply the case definition equally and without bias to all persons under investigation.

Methods for case finding will vary considerably according to the disease in question and the community setting. Most outbreaks involve certain clearly identifiable groups at risk; therefore, finding cases will be relatively self-evident and easy. Active, direct contact with selected physicians, hospitals, laboratories, schools, or industry or using some form of public announcement will find most of the remaining unreported cases. However, sometimes more intensive efforts—such as physician, telephone, door-to-door, culture, or serologic surveys—may be necessary to find cases. Regardless of the method, you must establish some system or systems of case finding during the investigation and perhaps afterwards (see Chapter 3).

Simply knowing the number of cases does not provide adequate information. Control and prevention measures depend upon knowing the source and mode of spread of an agent as well as the characteristics of ill patients. Therefore, case finding should include collecting pertinent information likely to provide clues or leads to the natural history of the epidemic and, particularly, relevant characteristics of the ill. First, collect basic information about each patient's age, gender, residence, occupation, and date of onset, for example, to define the basic descriptive aspects of the epidemic. Next, get pertinent signs, symptoms, and laboratory data. If the disease under investigation is usually water- or food-borne, ask questions about exposure to various water and food sources; if it is transmitted by person-to-person contact, ask about the frequency, duration, and nature of personal contacts. If the nature of the disease is not known or cannot be comfortably presumed, you will need to ask a variety of questions covering all possible aspects of disease transmission and risk. Also, be mentally prepared for the possibility of having to apply a second questionnaire if the first analysis does not help.

Orient the data in terms of time, place, and person

Now the team should have a reasonably accurate number of cases to view descriptively. So it is time to characterize the epidemic in terms of when patients became ill, where they lived or became ill, and what special attributes the patients had (see Chapter 6 for greater detail). You may want to wait until the epidemic is over or until all likely cases have been reported before performing such an analysis. Don't. The earlier you develop ideas of why the epidemic started, the more pertinent data you can collect. The addition of a proportionately small number of cases later on will usually not affect the analysis or recommendations.

Time.   Characterize the cases by plotting a graph that shows the number of cases (y axis) over the time of onset of illness using an appropriate time interval (x axis) (Figure 5–1). This "epidemic curve" gives a fairly deep appreciation for the magnitude of the outbreak, its possible mode of spread, and the possible duration of the epidemic—much more than would a simple "line listing" of cases. One can often infer a remarkable amount of information from a simple picture of times of onset of disease. If the incubation period of the disease is known, relatively firm inferences can be made regarding the likelihood of a point-source exposure, person-to-person spread, or a mixture of the two. Also, if the epidemic is in progress, you may be able to predict how many more cases are likely to occur. Finally, an epidemic curve provides an excellent "prop" for ready communication to nonepidemiologists, administrators, and the like who need to grasp in some fashion the nature and magnitude of the epidemic.

The epidemic curve in Figure 5–1 shows cases of Pontiac fever (subsequently confirmed as Legionnaires' disease) that occurred in Pontiac, Michigan, during July and August of 1968, by day of onset.[2] The epidemic was explosive in onset, suggesting (1) a virtually simultaneous common-source exposure of many persons, (2) a disease with a short incubation period, and (3) a continuing exposure spanning several weeks—all of which were subsequently verified.

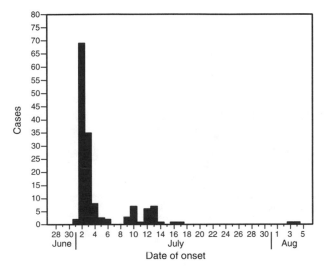

Figure 5-1.   Cases of Pontiac fever, by date of onset—Michigan, June 28-August 5, 1968.
Source: Glick et al. (1978).[2]

Place.   Sometimes diseases occur or are acquired in unique locations in the community, which, if you can visualize them may provide major clues or evidence regarding the source of the agent and/or the nature of exposure. Water supplies, milk distribution routes, sewage disposal outflows, prevailing wind currents, air-flow patterns in buildings, and ecologic habitats of vectors may play important roles in disseminating microbial or environmental pathogens and determining who is at risk of acquiring disease. If one plots cases geographically, a distribution pattern may appear that approximates these known sources and routes of potential exposure. This, in turn, may help identify the vehicle or mode of transmission.

Figure 5-2 illustrates the usefulness of a "spot map" in the investigation of an outbreak of shigellosis in Dubuque, Iowa, in 1974.[3] Early analysis showed that cases were not clustered by place of residence. A history of drinking water gave no useful clue as to a possible source and mode of transmission. However, it was later learned that many cases had been exposed to water by recent swimming in a camping park located on the Mississippi River. Figure 5-2 shows the river sites where 22 culture-positive cases swam within 3 days of onset of illness, strongly suggesting a common source of exposure. Ultimately, the epidemiologists incriminated Mississippi River water by documenting gross contamination by the city's sewage treatment plant 5 miles upstream and by isolating *Shigella sonnei* from a sample of river water taken from the camping park beach area.

Person.   Last, you must examine the characteristics of the patients themselves in terms of a variety of attributes, such as age, gender, race, occupation, or virtu-

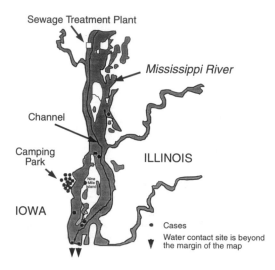

Figure 5-2. Culture-positive cases of shigellosis, by sites along the Mississippi River where each case swam within 3 days of onset of illness—Dubuque, Iowa, September 1974. *Source*: Rosenberg et al. (1976).[3]

ally any other characteristic that may be useful in portraying the uniqueness of the case population. If a singular or special attribute emerges, this frequently gives you a strong lead as to the group at risk and even an idea of the specific exposure. Some diseases primarily affect certain age groups or races; frequently, occupation is the key attribute of people with certain diseases. The list of human characteristics—really potential risks and exposures—is nearly endless. However, the more you know about the disease in question (the reservoir, mode or modes of spread, persons usually at greatest risk), the more specific and pertinent information you will have to determine whether any of these characteristics predisposes to illness.

Determine who is at risk of becoming ill

The field team now knows the number of people ill, when and where they were when they became ill, and what their general characteristics are; thus the team will usually have a firm diagnosis or a good "working" diagnosis. These data frequently provide enough information to determine with reasonable assurance how and why the epidemic started. For example, a time, place, and person description of the epidemic will strongly suggest that only people in a particular community supplied by a specific water system were at risk of getting sick, or that only certain students in a school or workers in a single factory became ill. Perhaps it was only a group of people who attended a local restaurant who reported illness. However, no matter how obvious it might appear that only a single group of persons was at risk, one should look carefully at the entire community to be sure there are no other affected persons.

Sometimes it is very difficult to know who is at risk. This is particularly true in epidemics that cover large geographic areas and involve many age groups with initially no obvious, unique characteristics. Under these circumstances, the team may have to do a survey of some kind to get more specific information about the ill persons and, hopefully, to get some idea of who is at risk.

Develop a hypothesis explaining the specific exposure that caused disease and test this hypothesis by appropriate statistical methods

This next step, the first real epidemiologic analysis of the field investigation, is often the most difficult one to perform. By now you should have an excellent grasp of the epidemic and an overall feel for the most likely source and mode of transmission. However, the exposure that caused disease must be determined.

A simple example is the 1989 investigation of an epidemic of nausea, vomiting, and diarrhea among 20 people who ate at a single pizzeria in McKeesport, Pennsylvania.[4] Since the disease was most likely acquired by eating something (because of the signs and symptoms) and since no other cluster of similar disease had occurred elsewhere in the community, the epidemiologists focused their attention only on those who bought food from the pizzeria. The logical hypothesis then was that the exposure necessary to develop nausea, vomiting, and diarrhea was consumption of some food or foods contaminated with a microbial or chemical agent. Therefore, those who bought and ate food from the pizzeria on the presumed day of exposure were given a questionnaire asking what beverages and kinds of foods and pizza they had eaten—that is, what foods had they been exposed to. Early analysis showed that 100 percent of the ill persons (cases) had eaten mushrooms on pizza. Because so many ill people ate these pizzas, one might quickly assume that the problem was the contaminated food. Yet the 100 percent finding simply represents how popular the mushroom pizza was among the ill attendees. Alone, it does not give adequate epidemiologic support to the hypothesis that the food exposure (i.e., eating the pizza) caused illness. What had to be done was to determine the food histories of the well pizza eaters (controls) and compare their histories to those of the ill persons. When this was done, the food histories were very similar between the two groups except for one food, the mushroom pizzas: only 33 percent of the well attendees ate the mushroom-topped pizza. The hypothesis, then, was that the difference in exposure rates—100 percent among the ill and 33 percent among the well—stemmed from mushroom pizza that was contaminated. When these different rates were compared and tested statistically, it was shown that such a difference would occur by chance less than once per 10,000 such instances if eating those pizzas was not related to disease. Therefore, the statistical evidence as well as other information (isolation of *S. aureus* from cans of mushrooms) supported the hypothesis that eating the mushroom pizza was the exposure necessary to produce illness.

Again, this phase of the investigation will clearly pose the greatest challenge. You must review the findings carefully; weigh the clinical, laboratory, and epidemiologic features of the disease; and hypothesize possible exposures that could plausibly cause illness. In other words, you must seek from the patients' histories exposures that could conceivably predispose to illness. If exposure histories for the ill and well are not significantly different, a new hypothesis must be developed. This will require imagination, perseverance, and sometimes the resurveying of those at risk to obtain more pertinent information.

Compare the hypothesis with the established facts

At this time in the investigation, epidemiologic and statistical inferences have provided the field team with data on the most probable exposure responsible for the epidemic. Yet you must "square" the hypothesis with the clinical, laboratory, and other epidemiologic facts of the investigation. In other words, do the proposed exposure, mode of spread, and population affected fit well with the known facts of the disease? For example, if, in the gastroenteritis outbreak referred to above, the analysis incriminated a food of high protein and low acid content that would support the growth of staphylococcal organisms and production of enterotoxin (as is the case with mushrooms), the hypothesis would fit well with our understanding of staphylococcal food poisoning. However, if the analysis incriminated coffee or water—highly unlikely sources of staphylococcal enterotoxin—you would then have to reassess the findings, perhaps secure more information, reconsider the clinical diagnosis, and certainly pose and test new hypotheses. Unfortunately, on rare occasions, this will happen, and one must be prepared.

The following investigations illustrate the uses of simple descriptive and analytic epidemiology, how some analyses may not prove helpful, how posing new hypotheses may be necessary, how the facts must fit logically, and how important persistence is in arriving at a defensible conclusion.

Between March 1 and September 1, 1981, in several maritime provinces of Canada, 34 cases of perinatal listeriosis and 7 cases of adult disease occurred.[5] These cases represented a severalfold increase over the number of cases diagnosed in previous years, suggesting some common exposure. Although *Listeria monocytogenes* is a common cause of abortion and nervous system disease in cattle, sheep, and goats, the source of human infection has been obscure. Cases could not be linked together by person-to-person contact; they shared no common water source; and food exposures, as determined from a general food history, were not different between cases and controls. However, a second, more detailed food history and subsequent intensive interrogation of cases and controls revealed that there was a statistically significant difference between cases and controls regarding exposure to coleslaw. Even though this food had never been previously incriminated as a source of *Listeria*, it was the only food item positively associated with disease and essentially the only lead the investigators had at the time. Armed with this clue, the team subsequently found a specimen of coleslaw in the refrigerator of one of the patients which grew out the same serotype of *Listeria* isolated from the epidemic cases. No other food items in the refrigerator were positive for *Listeria*.

The coleslaw had been prepared by a regional manufacturer who had obtained cabbages and carrots from several wholesale dealers and many local farmers. Although environmental cultures from the coleslaw plant failed to reveal *Listeria* organisms, two unopened packages of coleslaw from the plant subsequently grew *L. monocytogenes* of the same epidemic serotype. A review of the sources of the vegetable ingredients was made, and a single farmer was identified who had grown cabbages and also maintained a flock of sheep. Two of his sheep had previously died of listeriosis in 1979 and 1981. Also, he was in the habit of using sheep manure to fertilize his cabbages.

This information does not prove that this farm was the source of the *Listeria* organisms that caused the epidemic. However, the hypothesis that coleslaw was the source and the statistical test which supported this hypothesis provided the necessary impetus to continue the investigation. And, ultimately, a single, highly likely source of the bacteria was discovered. These findings strongly suggest that listeriosis is a zoonotic infection transmitted from infected animals via contaminated vegetables to humans.

In January and February 1980, an epidemic of 85 cases of salmonellosis in Ohio prompted an extensive field investigation by Taylor et al.[6] All were caused by an uncommon serotype of salmonella, *Salmonella meunchen*. This finding plus the fact that all cases were among teenagers and young adults strongly suggested a common source of exposure. Knowing that the natural reservoirs for almost all *Salmonella* serotypes are poultry, chicken eggs, and other domestic farm animals and that the majority of *Salmonella* epidemics can be traced to eating meat or poultry products or having contact with these animals, Taylor and colleagues questioned the cases and appropriate controls. Their questions included food histories and contact with farm animals. Not too surprisingly, the investigators found that significantly more cases gave a history of eating ham than did the controls. On the surface, this evidence strongly incriminated ham as the vehicle of infection. However, in trying to define the source of the contaminated ham, Taylor learned that the ham eaten by the patients came from five different distributors. How likely would it be for one uncommon serotype to come from five different distributors who, in turn, secured their ham from different producers? The logic was overwhelming: despite a reasonable food source of the *Salmonella* and persuasive statistics, the ham was not the source, and more questioning had to be done.

At this time another identical epidemic of *Salmonella* was reported in Michigan. Having more cases to work with and focusing on possible unique characteristics of the teenage/young adult population, the team asked many more questions of cases and controls, including questions about the use of drugs. To their great surprise, the epidemiologists found a highly significant association between illness and smoking marijuana. Although this association seemed just as implausible as that with the ham, samples of marijuana smoked by the cases were culture positive for *S. meunchen*, strongly incriminating the marijuana as the vehicle of infection.

Plan a more systematic study

The actual field investigation and analyses have now been completed, requiring only a written report (see below). However, because there may be a need to find more cases, to better define the extent of the epidemic, or to evaluate a new laboratory method or case-finding technique, you may want to perform more detailed and carefully executed studies. With the pressure of the investigation somewhat removed, consider surveying the population at risk in a variety of ways to help improve the quality of data and answer particular questions.

Perhaps the most important reasons to perform such studies are to improve the sensitivity and specificity of the case definition and establish more accurately the true number of persons at risk, (i.e., to improve the quality of numerators and denominators). For example, serosurveys coupled with more complete clinical histories can often sharpen the accuracy of the case count and define more clearly those truly at risk of developing disease. Moreover, repeated interviews of patients with confirmed disease may allow for rough quantitation of degrees of exposure or dose responses—useful information in understanding the pathogenesis of certain diseases.

Prepare a written report

Frequently, the team's final responsibility is to prepare a written report to document the investigation, the findings, and the recommendations (see Chapter 11). There are several important reasons why a report should be written and as soon as possible.

A Document for Action.   Sometimes control and prevention efforts will only be taken when a report of all relevant findings has been written. This can and should place a heavy but necessary burden on the field team to complete their work quickly. Even if all possible cases have not yet been found or some laboratory results are still pending, reasonable written assumptions and recommendations can usually be made without fear of retraction or subsequent major change.

A Record of Performance.   In this day of input and output measurements, program planning, program justifications, and performance evaluations, there is often no better record of accomplishment than a well-written report of a completed field investigation. The number of investigations performed and the time and re-sources expended not only document the magnitude of health problems, changes in disease trends, and results of control and prevention efforts but also serve as concrete evidence of program justification and needs.

A Document for Potential Medical/Legal Issues.   Presumably, epidemiolo-gists investigate epidemics with objective, unbiased, and scientific purposes and similarly prepare written reports of their findings and conclusions objectively, hon-estly, and fairly. Such information may prove absolutely invaluable to consum-ers, practicing physicians, or local and state health department officials in any legal action regarding health responsibilities and jurisdictions (see Chapter 14). In the long run, the health of the public is best served by the simple, careful, honest documentation of events and findings, which are made available for interpreta-tion and comment.

Enhancement of the Quality of the Investigation.   Although not fully under-stood and rarely referred to, the actual process of writing and viewing data in writ-ten form often generates new and different thought processes and associations in one's mind (see Chapter 10). The discipline of committing to paper the clinical, laboratory, and epidemiologic findings of an epidemic investigation will almost always bring to light not only a better understanding of the natural unfolding of events but also of their importance in terms of the natural history and development of the epidemic. The actual process of creating scientific prose, summarizing data, and creating tables and figures representing the known, established facts forces the epidemiologist to view the entire series of events in a balanced, rational, and ex-plainable way. These characteristics are considerably more marked than they would be in an oral report given to the local health department the day of departure from the field. Occasionally, previously unrecognized associations will emerge from a careful, step-by-step written analysis, and this may be critical in the final interpre-tation and recommendations. The exercise of writing what was done and what was found will sometimes uncover facts and events that were more or less assumed to be true but not specifically sought for during the investigation. This, in turn, may stimulate further inquiry and fact finding in order to verify these assumptions.

An Instrument for Teaching Epidemiology.   There would hardly be disagree-ment among epidemiologists that the exercise of writing the results of an investi-gation constitutes an essential building block in learning epidemiology. Much the way a lawyer prepares a brief, the epidemiologist should know how to organize and present in logical sequence the important and pertinent findings of an investigation, their quality and validity, and the scientific inferences that can be made by their written presentation. The simple, direct, and orderly array of facts and inferences will reflect not only the quality of the investigation itself but also the writer's basic understanding and knowledge of the epidemiologic method.

Execute control and prevention measures

It is not the purpose of this chapter to discuss this aspect of a field investigation. Nevertheless, the underlying purposes of all epidemic investigations are to control and/or prevent further disease.

SUMMARY

In sum, the field investigation is a direct application of the epidemiologic method, very often with an implied and relatively circumscribed timetable. This forces you to (1) establish workable case-finding techniques, (2) collect data rapidly but carefully, and (3) describe cases in a general sense regarding the time and place of occurrence and those primarily affected. Usually, you will know the agent and its sources and modes of transmission, which will allow you to identify the source and mode of spread rapidly. However, when the clinical disease is obscure and/or the origin of the agent ill defined, you may be hard-pressed to create a hypothesis that will not only identify the critical exposure and show statistical significance but also logically explain the occurrence of the epidemic. Although you will not be able to prove, scientifically, causation in the strictest sense, in most instances the careful development of epidemiologic inferences, coupled with persuasive clinical and laboratory data, will almost always provide convincing evidence of why the epidemic occurred. Last, a written report will not only serve to sharpen your communication and epidemiologic skills but also provide the health community with permanent documentation of your investigation.

REFERENCES

1. Centers for Disease Control and Prevention (1977). Unpublished data.
2. Glick, T. H., Gregg, M. B., Berman, B., et al. (1978). Pontiac fever: An epidemic of unknown etiology in a health department: I. Clinical and epidemiological aspects. *American Journal of Epidemiology*, 107, 149–60.
3. Rosenberg, M. D., Hazlet, K. K., Schaefer, J., et al. (1976). Shigellosis from swimming. *Journal of the American Medical Association*, 236, 1849–52.

4. Centers for Disease Control (1989). Multiple outbreaks of staphylococcal food poisoning caused by canned mushrooms. *Morbidity and Mortality Weekly Report*, 38, 417–18.
5. Schlech, W. F. III, Lavigne, P. M., Bortobussi, R. A., et al. (1983). Epidemic listeriosis—Evidence for transmission by food. *New England Journal of Medicine*, 308, 203–206.
6. Taylor, D. N., Wachsmith, K., Shangkuan, Y., et al. (1982). Salmonellosis associated marijuana: A multistate outbreak traced by plasmid fingerprinting. *New England Journal of Medicine*, 306, 1249–53.

6

DESCRIBING EPIDEMIOLOGIC DATA

Richard A. Goodman
J. Virgil Peavy

One of the most basic and important tasks an epidemiologist faces is organizing and describing data. This task is sometimes called *descriptive epidemiology*, which addresses the questions *how much* (e.g., how much disease is occurring), *when*, *where*, and *to whom*. In epidemiology, the last three of these dimensions are usually referred to as *time*, *place*, and *person*. Characterizing epidemiologic data along these dimensions serves several purposes. First, this approach provides a systematic method for dissecting a health event or problem into its fundamental components, and it ensures that you are familiar with the basic dimensions of that health event or problem. Second, the approach provides a detailed characterization of the problem in basic terms that can easily be communicated and understood. Third, it identifies populations at increased risk of the health problem under investigation, enabling you then to generate testable hypotheses relevant to etiology, mode of spread, and other aspects of the problem. This epidemiologic sequence is analogous to the diagnostic sequence of the clinician, who first obtains baseline data from the history and physical examination before the diagnosis can be hypothesized and evaluated by using specific tests.

This chapter outlines some of the key concepts in descriptive epidemiology, and presents an approach to the characterization of epidemiologic data. Guidelines for using graphs and charts in descriptive epidemiology are presented in Appendix 6–1 at the end of this chapter.

The extent to which a health problem can be characterized by time, place, and person may be a function of the initial database. For example, outbreak investigations usually rely on "line listings," a detailed list of cases, line by line, including demographic features, occupation, special activities, and many other variables. In contrast, routine surveillance databases contain considerably less information, perhaps little more than date of report, residence, age, and gender.

HOW MUCH DISEASE?

The simplest way to determine the extent of a health event is to count cases. As noted in earlier chapters, counts can be compared to historical norms in order to look for unusual patterns and outbreaks. However, simple case counts are often insufficient for epidemiologic purposes. Suppose the number of persons seriously injured while rollerblading this year was double the number injured last year. Has rollerblading become more dangerous? Similarly, suppose that, in the past month, an urban county had twice the number of hepatitis A cases as did a rural county. Is the urban dweller more likely to contract hepatitis A than the rural resident?

Those questions are not answerable from the data provided. To assess the issue of risk, the numbers of cases must be placed in proper perspective. That is, the number of cases must be assessed in light of the size of the population from which they arose. Rates are measures for relating cases to the population. With rates, you can determine whether one group or another is at increased risk of disease, and by how much. From a population perspective, these so-called high-risk groups can be further assessed and targeted for special intervention. From an individual perspective, by comparing rates, you may also identify risk factors for disease. Identification of these risk factors may be used by individuals in their day-to-day decision making about behaviors that influence their health.

A variety of measures are used in epidemiology to quantify the occurrence or presence of adverse health events.

Mortality and Morbidity Rates

Mortality rates describe the occurrence of death in a population. Morbidity rates describe the frequency of illness within a population. For both mortality and morbidity measures, the time and place must be specified.

The most commonly used morbidity measures in field epidemiology are *incidence rate*, *attack rate*, and *prevalence*.

Incidence rate

Incidence measures the rapidity with which a health condition develops or the frequency with which new cases are occurring in a population. The numerator is the number of new cases. The denominator is the size of the population from which these cases arose. Incidence is always calculated for a given period of time.

Attack rate

An *attack rate* is the proportion of a well-defined population that develops illness over a limited period of time, as during an epidemic or outbreak. The numerator is the number of new cases that occurred during that time period. The denominator is the size of the population at risk at the start of the time period. It is often expressed as a percentage.

Prevalence

Prevalence measures the proportion of the population that has a particular condition or attribute. The numerator includes both new and preexisting cases. Point prevalence represents the proportion of the population that has a particular condition or attribute at a given instant in time (e.g., the number of cases of diabetes in a given city on July 1, 1994). Period prevalence represents the proportion of the population that has a particular condition or attribute during a specified period of time (e.g., the number of persons who were seropositive for the human immunodeficiency virus over the year 1994 in the same city). Incidence is most useful for measuring acute events such as infectious diseases (e.g., the number of measles cases reported in New York during the week of April 2 to 8, 1994). Prevalence, on the other hand, gives the most useful information on conditions of a long-term or chronic nature (e.g., the number of persons with tuberculosis in Peoria, Illinois, in 1994).

TIME

In looking at epidemiologic data, you must always consider the element of time. For example, as noted above, morbidity and mortality rates require that you specify the relevant time period. Similarly, the assessment of an outbreak requires that you compare the number of cases during a specific time period to the expected number for that time period. When you consider time, you need to address the pertinent time period or periods, the temporal relation between exposure and health events, the display of time data, and examination of the data.

Time Periods

Depending on the health event you are studying, the time period of interest may include many years or may be limited to a period during which the reported number of cases exceeds the expected or usual number of cases for that period (an epidemic period). For some conditions, including many chronic diseases, the time characteristic of interest is the secular trend—the annual number or rate of disease over many years. For other conditions, a description by season, month, day of the week, or even time of day may be revealing. Periodic changes, such as seasonal variations, may be more characteristic of problems that occur in regular or predictable cycles. For example, the incidence of varicella appears to be seasonal, since outbreaks tend to occur between March and May (Figure 6–1).[1] For newly recognized problems, time should be assessed in a variety of ways to determine the most appropriate and revealing characterizations.

Temporal Relation between Exposure and Occurrence

To the extent possible, both the time of exposure to risk factors and the time of onset of the health event should be determined. When the etiology is unknown, the interval between time of presumed exposure and time of onset of symptoms is critical in hypothesizing the etiology, since it allows you to estimate incubation or latency periods.

Relevant events should be placed in temporal sequence to help create an accurate chronologic framework for investigating the problem. Time of occurrence should be determined or estimated for the following events:

- Time or period(s) of exposure to risk factors/causal agents
- Onset of manifestations in cases and contacts
- Treatments, implementation of control measures, or other interventions
- Time of potentially related events or unusual circumstances

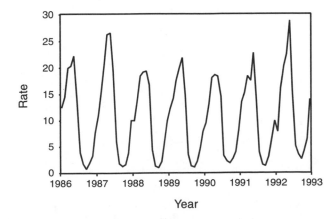

Figure 6–1. Rate (reported cases per 100,000 population) of varicella (chickenpox)–United States, 1986–1992. *Source:* CDC (1992).[1]

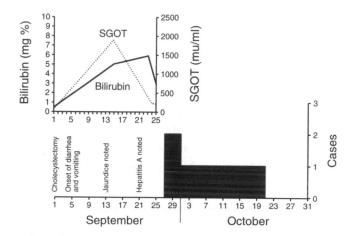

Figure 6–2.   Correlation of hospital course of hepatitis A source patient with laboratory values and onset of illness in secondary cases—Georgia, September 1–October 31, 1980. *Source:* Goodman et al. (1982).[2]

These principles are illustrated in Figure 6–2, which shows the hospital course of a patient who was admitted for an elective cholecystectomy but was incubating hepatitis A at that time.[2] Six secondary cases occurred in hospital staff who cared for the source case and another in her hospital roommate. In Figure 6–3, the incidence of malaria in the United States is shown for the period 1930–1992 in relation to important events that have accounted for trends in malaria occurrence.[3]

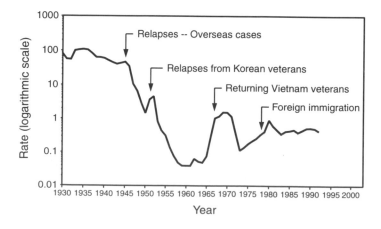

Figure 6–3.   Rate (reported cases per 100,000 population) of malaria—United States, 1930–1992. *Source:* CDC (1992).[3]

Sometimes it may be useful to describe health events by time of onset of manifestations, including symptoms, signs, or positive diagnostic tests. The accuracy of this information can vary considerably by problem and may be greater for acute problems that have occurred recently than for those which are chronic in nature. If you know both the time of onset and the time of known or presumed exposure, you can then estimate the incubation or latency period. Determining the time of onset in secondary cases also helps you establish the incubation or latency period. Examination of the time that elapses between the occurrence of cases and implementation of control measures may help you to generate hypotheses concerning etiology, mode of spread, and effectiveness of measures. Identification of special events or unusual circumstances temporally related to the problem may also help in the formulation of relevant hypotheses. For certain types of problems, the time of precipitating events must be carefully distinguished from time of occurrence of the outcome (e.g., injury and death).

How to Graph Time Data

Time data are usually displayed graphically. The number or rate of cases or deaths is specified along the y axis; the time intervals are specified along the x axis. The graph may indicate the timing of events thought to be related to the health problem, such as the period of exposure or the date of implementation of a control measure. The purpose of this graph is to provide a simple visual depiction of the relative magnitude, past trends, and potential future course of the problem and the impact of specified related events. The graph may also suggest hypotheses concerning causes.

Number of Cases over Time

Traditionally, the number of cases of a health event over time are graphed with a histogram. If the time period of interest represents the duration of an epidemic, the histogram is called an *epidemic curve*. The number of cases is specified on the y axis, while the time intervals are specified on the x axis. In general, the time intervals used on the x axis should be less than the known or suspected incubation/latency period; by convention, the time intervals may be approximately one-fourth to one-third the probable incubation period.

To assess whether time of onset (or exposure) varies in relation to place or person characteristics, epidemic curves may be constructed that stratify case groups by place (e.g., residence, employment, or school) or by personal characteristics (e.g., age, gender, race, etc.).

Rates over Time

Whereas numbers of cases over time are usually graphed with a histogram, rates of disease over time are usually graphed with a line graph or frequency polygon. The x axis represents the period of time in which you are interested: decades, years, months, day of the week, or even time of day. The y axis represents the rate of the health event per 1,000, per 100,000, or whatever is appropriate for the event. For most conditions, the rates vary over one or two orders of magnitude, so an arithmetic scale is appropriate. For rates that vary more widely and/or when comparisons are made, a semilogarithmic scale may be more appropriate.

Special Features

Specific labels should be used to designate cases with unique importance (e.g., those suspected of introducing the problem or playing an essential role in propagation of the problem), to indicate the occurrence of special events related to the problem, and to reflect the implementation of control measures. For example, Figure 6–4 shows an epidemic curve of salmonellosis in airline passengers who were en route from London to Los Angeles and had been served contaminated meals during the flight.[4]

Examining Your Graphs

Epidemic curves

Examination of the epidemic curve may provide you with an estimate of the relative magnitude of the problem and may suggest hypotheses concerning the origin of the problem, the source and mode of spread of the etiologic agent, and the nature of the etiologic agent and its incubation or latency period. In addition, extrapolation from the epidemic curve may help you predict the end of an outbreak or help you project the occurrence of additional cases.

The configuration of the epidemic curve often suggests the nature of the etiologic agent as well as its source and mode of spread. Distortions in the case-time relation that are associated with use of inappropriate time intervals may mislead you about the source or mode of spread. In particular, you should use a time interval that is less than the known or suspected incubation period so as to reduce the likelihood that person-to-person spread is misclassified as common-source spread. Figures 6–5A and 6–5B demonstrate the effects of the time scale on the appearance of an epidemic curve. Both curves show the same measles outbreak, usually transmitted through person-to-person spread.[5] Note in Figure 6–5A that measles cases are plotted by day of onset, showing three separate peaks of cases.

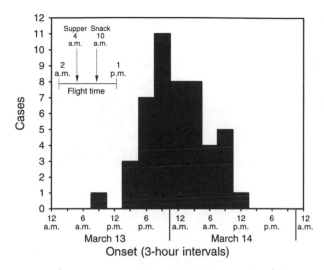

Figure 6–4.   Salmonellosis in passengers on a flight from London to the United States, by time of onset, March 13–14, 1984. *Source:* Tauxe et al. (1987).[4]

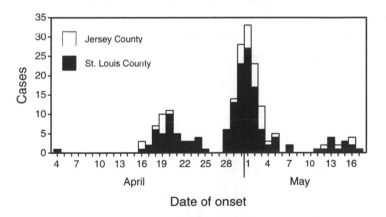

Figure 6–5A.   Measles cases, by date of rash onset and location—St. Louis County, Missouri, and Jersey County, Illinois, April 4–May 17, 1994. *Source:* CDC (1994).[5]

The times between peaks roughly equal the incubation period of measles—all of which suggest person-to-person transmission. Figure 6–5B shows the same data; however, cases are plotted by week of onset. Here the visual impression is totally different. Instead of three peaks, there is only one, suggesting a common source exposure.

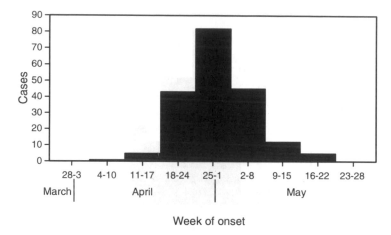

Figure 6–5B. Measles cases, by week of onset of rash—St. Louis County, Missouri, and Jersey County, Illinois, April 4–May 17, 1994. *Source:* CDC (1994).[5]

Point source

An epidemic curve that shows a relatively tight temporal clustering of cases, a sharp upslope, and a gentler downslope is consistent with a point source for the agent. A point source is a common vehicle, such as a food or beverage, to which persons have been exposed for only one well-defined, relatively brief period of time. Figure 6–6 shows an epidemic curve for a Norwalk viral gastroenteritis outbreak following contamination of a community water system and temporally related exposure to the water.[6]

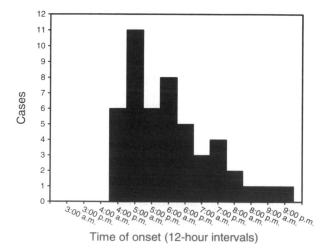

Figure 6–6. Cases of gastrointestinal illness in persons living in households served by the Tate community water supply—Georgia, January 13, 1982. *Source:* Goodman et al. (1982).[6]

Person to person

An epidemic curve exhibiting a clustering of cases but characterized by a relatively gentle upslope and somewhat steeper tail suggests that an infectious agent has been transmitted from person to person. An outbreak of type B influenza in a nursing home illustrates these features (Figure 6–7).[7] A second but less prominent cluster of cases might indicate secondary transmission from person to person when an infectious agent is responsible.

Intermittent or continuing common source

When the epidemic curve shows the occurrence of individual or clustered cases over a relatively protracted time period, either an intermittent or continuing common source of the agent is suggested. The occurrence of more prominent case clusters during the time period might reflect secondary person-to-person transmission if an infectious agent is implicated.

Vector-borne disease

In general, the epidemic curves of arthropod-borne diseases start slowly, have irregular peaks, and slowly tail away. The curve may extend over weeks or months (Figure 6–8).[8]

The incubation period may be estimated by examining the duration between the time of known or presumed exposure to the peak of the epidemic curve. This may help you identify the etiologic agent when it is otherwise unknown. For ex-

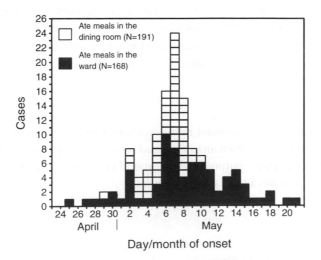

Figure 6–7. Cases of influenzalike illness among nursing home residents, by date of onset and patient's dining area—rural Minnesota, April 24–May 21, 1979. *Source:* Hall et al. (1981).[7]

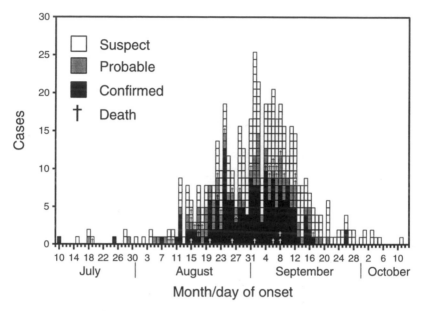

Figure 6-8. Cases of St. Louis encephalitis–Chicago standard metropolitan statistical area, July 10–October 12, 1975. *Source:* CDC (1975).[8]

ample, when an apparently short incubation period accompanies an epidemic curve with a steep upslope, this suggests a point-source exposure to an infectious or toxic agent. Cases that occur either very early or substantially later relative to an outbreak should be carefully examined for clues suggesting etiology, source, or mode of spread. For problems of infectious etiology, the earliest cases should be considered as potential *source* cases. Early and late cases, sometimes called *outliers*, may give very useful leads if examined carefully.

Rates

The determination of background rates—rates that occur under normal circumstances and are available from an established surveillance system—can serve as a baseline for comparative purposes. Background rates can also assist in forecasting trends for diseases and health conditions.

PLACE

The second dimension of descriptive epidemiology is place. Characterizing epidemiologic data by place documents the geographic extent of the health problem and may help you develop hypotheses concerning location of exposure.

Information on Place

During investigations of outbreaks or acute problems, you may want to obtain information that relates place to affected persons, including place of residence (e.g., by census tract), employment, school, recreation, recent travel, or other relevant categories. You may need to collect data of greater specificity to describe activities further in these locations, such as information detailing movement within a building or office suite and determining the duration of time spent in a given location.

For some problems, descriptive epidemiology may focus more appropriately on the broader geographic distribution of that problem. Geographic parameters to be examined might include occurrence of the problem in relation to natural boundaries and topography; statutory and geopolitical demarcations (such as state boundaries or county lines); climate, different weather patterns, or latitudes; and other ecologic or environmental determinants.

How to Examine Place

In outbreak investigations, cases can be plotted to develop a "spot map" by using a map or, for very specific locations, a diagram such as a floor plan, where ill persons (cases) are depicted by their places of employment, residence, or other locations. In addition, epidemic curves can be constructed that segregate cases based on different places. These approaches may then lead to the development of specific hypotheses concerning the location of a reservoir for the etiologic agent or the site or sites of transmission. For example, the epidemic curve of the Norwalk virus outbreak in Figure 6–9 demonstrates that onsets of illness varied in terms of place and times of exposure to the agent.[9] Persons who lived in the community were exposed to the contaminated system (over the weekend) before many of the students who resided elsewhere but attended school in that community. When larger geographic areas are examined, shading or other techniques can be used to contrast rates of occurrence in different areas.

Regardless of the thrust of the investigation, however, you should always attempt to distinguish between place of onset and place of exposure; while they may be the same, they are often different.

PERSON

The purposes of examining epidemiologic data in terms of person are to thoroughly describe the case group and identify features shared in common by the cases. Rigorous description of the case population will help you develop hypotheses

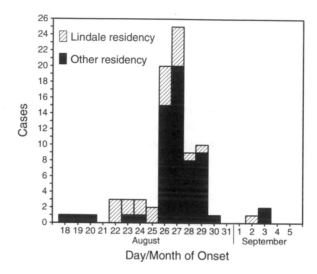

Figure 6–9.   Cases of gastroenteritis among junior and senior high school students, by date of onset and residency—Lindale area of Rome, Georgia, August 18–September 3, 1980. *Source:* Kaplan et al. (1982).[9]

concerning host characteristics that may constitute risk factors, other potential risk factors, and the source and mode of spread of the agent.

Attribute Categories

The cases may be characterized by several categories of attributes: demographic characteristics of those affected (including age, race/ethnic group, and gender), socioeconomic status, education, occupation, leisure activities, religion, marital status, contact with other persons or groups, and other personal variables (such as pregnancy, blood type, immunization status, underlying illnesses, or use of medications).

Examination of Person Data

Information on person can be presented in either tabular form or graphically. Tabular presentation may be as basic as univariate frequency distributions or as complex as necessary to indicate frequencies relative to other key variables.

Interpretation of Person Data

Two important qualifications apply to the interpretation of person data. First, the risk of developing illness can be estimated only by the use of specific denominators and thus requires that you determine rates. Second, age is one of the strongest independent determinants for many causes of morbidity and mortality and, accordingly, deserves great consideration. Figure 6–10 shows the distribution of farm tractor–related fatalities in Georgia by age group of the decedent.[10] Age group–specific fatality rates derived by using two different denominator groups are listed in Table 6–1.

Table 6–1. Annual Fatality Rates per 100,000 Males in Accidents Associated with Farm Tractors, Georgia, 1971–1981

AGE GROUP (YEARS)	NUMBER OF DEATHS	FARM RESIDENTS		ALL RURAL RESIDENTS	
		RATE	STANDARD ERROR	RATE	STANDARD ERROR
<20	21	6.7	± 1.5	0.5	± 0.1
20–39	32	22.3	± 4.0	1.1	± 0.2
40–59	65	27.6	± 3.4	3.1	± 0.4
≥ 60	80	54.1	± 6.1	6.4	± 0.1
Total	198	23.6		1.9	

Source: Goodman et al. (1992).[10]

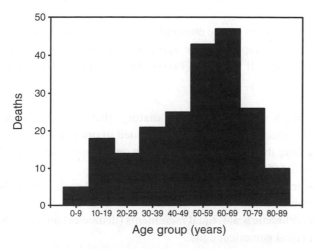

Figure 6–10. Deaths associated with farm tractor accidents, by age group—Georgia, 1971–1991. *Source:* Goodman et al. (1992).[10]

SUMMARY

In summary, descriptive epidemiology includes both numbers and rates to document how much of a health condition is present or occurring in a population. The three critical dimensions for describing a health condition are time, place, and person. *Time* can refer to acute changes in disease occurrence, such as an epidemic, seasonal patterns, and secular trends. Time data are usually displayed graphically. *Place* can refer to geopolitical boundaries, topography, or location of rooms, buildings, and other structures. Place data are usually displayed with maps. *Person* refers to demographic and other personal characteristics of the populations under study. Person data are usually displayed in tables or graphs. When done well, descriptive epidemiology can characterize the health problem in a community, provide clues that can be turned into testable hypotheses, and promote effective communication with scientific, policymaking, and lay audiences alike.

APPENDIX 6-1. GRAPHS AND CHARTS IN DESCRIPTIVE EPIDEMIOLOGY

GENERAL PRINCIPLES

When graphs have been drawn correctly, they should give the viewer a rapid, objective, overall grasp of the data. Some of the most important principles of graphing are outlined below.

The simplest graphs are the most effective. No more lines or symbols should be used in a single graph than the eye can easily follow or than the viewer can easily understand. If more than two or three points are to be made, use two graphs.

- Every graph should be self-explanatory; that is, it should be titled and labeled correctly so that no text is needed to orient the viewer.
- When more than one variable is shown on a graph, each should be clearly differentiated by means of legends or keys.
- Frequency is usually represented on the vertical scale and method of classification on the horizontal scale.
- On an arithmetic scale, equal increments (distances) on the scale must represent equal numerical units.
- Scale divisions should be clearly indicated, as well as the units into which the scale is divided.

ALTERNATIVE APPROACHES FOR GRAPHING TIME

Two options for displaying and assessing epidemiologic rates include arithmetic and semilog graphs.

Arithmetic Scale Line Graph

In a scale line graph, an equal distance on the y axis represents an equal quantity anywhere on a given axis. Judgment is required to determine whether to use equal intervals on both axes, wide intervals on the x axis in relation to the y axis, or vice versa. The scales should be defined in such a way as to make it easy to understand. When possible, a break in the scale should not be used with a scale line graph. Figure 6–11 is an example of an arithmetic scale line graph.[11]

Semilogarithmic Scale Line Graph

In a semilogarithmic scale line graph, one coordinate or axis (usually the y axis) is measured in logarithms of units, whereas the other axis is measured in arithmetic units. This approach may be useful for examining the relative rate of change rather than the absolute change (i.e., actual amount of change). It is particularly helpful when comparing two or more variables whose rates are different by large orders of magnitude. The advantages of semilog graphing are that (1) a straight

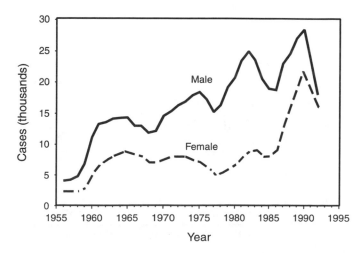

Figure 6–11.   Reported cases of primary and secondary syphilis, by gender—United States, 1956–1992. *Source:* CDC (1992).[11]

line indicates a constant rate of change, (2) the slope of the line indicates the rate of increase or decrease, (3) two or more lines following parallel paths show identical rates of increase (or decrease), and (4) a wide range of values (three to four orders of magnitude) can be displayed effectively on a single graph. An illustration of this type of graph is shown by the larger graph of Figure 6–12.[12]

HISTOGRAMS

A histogram is a graph used to present the frequency distribution of quantitative data and, in the context of an outbreak investigation, is often referred to as an *epidemic curve* (see above). On a histogram, adjacent columns are not separated by space. In comparison, on a bar chart, columns are separated by spaces. A scale break should not be used in the histogram because the histogram depicts the total area under the curve. Because of this characteristic, the easiest type of histogram to construct will be one of equal class intervals, as shown in Figure 6–13.[13]

For illustration, Figure 6–13 shows the area under the curve partitioned into each case of illness. In general, only the line representing the height of each column is drawn. To ensure that the area of each rectangle in the histogram represents a specified number of cases, the height represents the number of cases per unit of measurement (in Figure 6–13, per day) and the width, the method of classification (in Figure 6–13, interval of time in days). Therefore, the product of the height and width will equal the number of cases within a day.

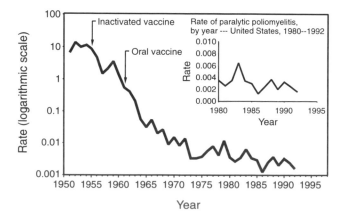

Figure 6–12. Rate (reported cases per 100,000 population) of paralytic poliomyelitis—United States, 1951–1992. *Source:* CDC (1992).[12]

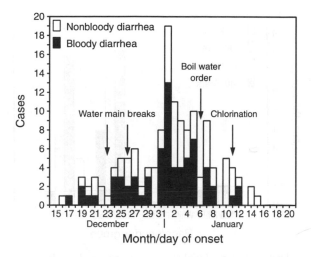

Figure 6–13. Cases of diarrheal illness in city residents, by date of onset and character of stool—Cabool, Missouri, December 1989–January 1990. *Source:* CDC (1990).[13]

CHARTS

Charts are methods of presenting statistical information symbolically using only one coordinate. Charts presented here include those based on length and proportion.

Bar Charts

In a bar chart, all cells are characterized by an identical column width. In addition, in contrast to a histogram, columns are separated by spaces. Bar charts are ideally suited for presenting comparative data. The bars may be arrayed horizontally as well as vertically, as illustrated in Figure 6–14, and should be arranged in either ascending or descending order for ease of reading.[14] Scale breaks should never be used in bar charts. However, columns may be shaded, hatched, or colored to emphasize differences between the bars. To ensure simplicity, the bars should be labeled at the bottom and not in the middle of the chart. When comparisons are made, the space between bars in the same group is optional, but space between groups is mandatory.

Pie Charts

Pie charts use wedge-shaped portions of a circle to facilitate comparisons. The pie chart is best adapted for illustrating the division of the whole into segments. By convention, begin at the 12 o'clock position and arrange segments in order of

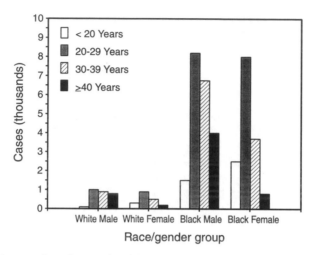

Figure 6–14.   Number of cases of syphilis, by age, race, and gender–United States, 1989. *Source:* CDC (1989).[14]

magnitude—largest first, then proceeding clockwise around the chart. To convert from percentage to degrees, multiply the percentage by 3.6, since $360°/100 = 3.6°$. Figures 6–15[15] and 6–16[16] are examples of pie charts.

SUGGESTIONS FOR THE DESIGN AND USE OF TABLES, GRAPHS, AND CHARTS

- Choose the tool that is most effective for data and purpose. First specify the point that must be communicated, then choose the method. Continuous line graphs are suitable for a comparison of trends; bar charts clearly compare separate quantities of limited number; and pie charts have advantages in comparing parts to their whole. Do not forget with whom you are communicating. Lay audiences (including policymakers, administrators, etc.) will understand you much better if you choose the simplest of presentations.
- Emphasize one idea at a time. Confine the presentation to one purpose or idea. Limit the amount of data and include only one kind of datum in each presentation.
- Use adequate and properly located labels. Titles should include the "what, where, and when" that completely identify the data they introduce. All other labels should be equally clear, complete, and easy to understand. Like the title, they should be outside the frame of the data. Only keys or legends should appear within the field of a graph or chart. Keys and legends should be clearly distinguished from the data.

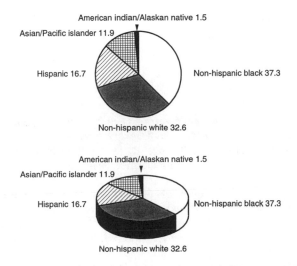

Figure 6-15. Percentage of tuberculosis cases, by race/ethnicity—United States, 1989. *Source:* CDC (1989).[15]

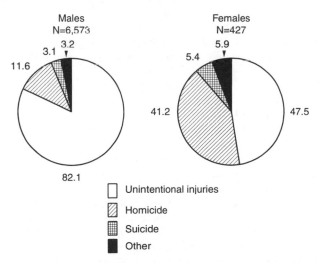

Figure 6-16. Percentage of traumatic deaths among workers, by gender and cause of death—United States, 1980-1985. *Source:* CDC (1985).[16]

- Provide sources. The source of the data should be provided. Verification or further analysis by the audience is difficult or impossible without full disclosure of sources.
- Base conclusions on the data. Conclusions should reflect the full body of information from which data were excerpted. Note, however, that tables, graphs, and charts emphasize generalities. Thus, potential distortions should

be compensated for both in design and in comment by using footnotes or other means to note important detail that has been obscured.

REFERENCES

1. Centers for Disease Control and Prevention (1992). Summary of notifiable diseases, United States. *Morbidity and Mortality Weekly Report*, 41, 64.
2. Goodman, R. A., Carder, C. C., Allen, J. R., et al. (1982). Nosocomial hepatitis A: Transmission by an adult patient with diarrhea. *American Journal of Medicine*, 73, 220–26.
3. Centers for Disease Control and Prevention (1992). Summary of notifiable diseases, United States. *Morbidity and Mortality Weekly Report*, 41, 38.
4. Tauxe, R. V., Tormey, M. P., Mascola, L., et al. (1987). Salmonellosis outbreak in transatlantic flights; Foodborne illness on aircraft: 1947–1984. *American Journal of Epidemiology*, 125, 150–57.
5. Centers for Disease Control and Prevention (1994). Outbreak of measles among Christian Science students—Missouri and Illinois, 1994. *Morbidity and Mortality Weekly Report*, 43, 463–65.
6. Goodman, R. A., Buehler, J. W., Greenberg, H. B., et al. (1982). Norwalk gastroenteritis associated with a water system in a rural Georgia community. *Archives of Environmental Health*, 37, 358–60.
7. Hall, W. N., Goodman, R. A., Noble, G. R., et al. (1981). An outbreak of influenza B in an elderly population. *Journal of Infectious Diseases*, 144, 190–97.
8. Centers for Disease Control (1975). Unpublished data.
9. Kaplan, J. E., Goodman, R. A., Schonberger, L. B., et al. (1982). Gastroenteritis due to Norwalk virus: An outbreak associated with a municipal water system. *Journal of Infectious Diseases*, 146, 190–97.
10. Goodman, R. A., Smith, J. D., Sikes, R. K., et al. (1992). An epidemiologic study of fatalities associated with farm tractor injuries. *Public Health Reports*, 100, 329–33.
11. Centers for Disease Control and Prevention (1992). Summary of notifiable diseases, United States, 1992. *Morbidity and Mortality Weekly Report*, 41, 55.
12. Centers for Disease Control and Prevention (1992). Summary of notifiable diseases, United States, 1992. *Morbidity and Mortality Weekly Report*, 41, 46.
13. Centers for Disease Control and Prevention (1990). Unpublished data.
14. Centers for Disease Control and Prevention (1989). Unpublished data.
15. Centers for Disease Control and Prevention (1989). Summary of notifiable diseases, United States, 1989. *Morbidity and Mortality Weekly Report*, 38, 45.
16. Centers for Disease Control, National Institute for Occupational Safety and Health (1985). Unpublished data.

7

DESIGNING STUDIES IN THE FIELD

James W. Buehler
Richard C. Dicker

For all but the most straightforward field investigations, the epidemiologist is likely to design and conduct an epidemiologic study of some sort. Such a study is an efficient mechanism to evaluate hypotheses that have been raised in earlier phases of the investigation. Its hallmark is a comparison group that provides baseline or "expected" data. By comparing the observed data with the expected data from the comparison group, you can quantify the relationship between possible risk factors and disease and can test the statistical significance of various hypotheses.

In an experimental study, such as a therapeutic trial, a group of study participants is selected, randomly allocated into exposure and control groups, and then monitored. In public health practice, however, epidemiologists usually cannot conduct experiments to test the relationship between exposures and diseases. Instead, we rely on observational study designs to make comparisons between different groups of people and to assess associations between exposures and health outcomes.

There are two basic types of epidemiologic studies in which comparisons are made. In one approach, the occurrence of disease is compared for persons who are or are not exposed to a risk factor (cohort or follow-up study). In the other, past exposures are compared in persons who do and do not have a disease (case-control study). Conceptually, the cohort design is generally more straightforward than the case-control design as a technique to relate exposures to disease outcomes. But the case-control design is often the more expedient approach when one is confronted with an acute problem and an urgent need to identify possible etiologies.

This chapter provides an overview of these two study approaches, emphasizing methodologic considerations in the field. For more in-depth discussion of these issues, the reader is referred to standard epidemiology texts.[1,2]

Defining Exposed and Unexposed Groups

Since both cohort and case-control studies are used to quantify exposure-disease relationships, it is critical to define clearly what is meant by "exposure" and by "disease". In situations where the exposure is a relatively discrete event, defining exposure status is conceptually straightforward, (i.e., defining who did or did not eat a certain food, or who was or was not acutely exposed to a toxic agent in a chemical spill). Exposures can be subdivided by dose or duration and can be combined in a variety of ways ("ate any item with mayonnaise"). "Exposure" can also refer to host characteristics, such as age, gender, or ABO blood type.

In other situations, exposures may be prolonged and difficult to quantify. Examples include diseases resulting from prolonged exposures such as passively inhaled cigarette smoke, chronic dietary patterns, or low doses of radiation. In some cases, exposures may be ongoing and may influence the risk of further complications once disease has occurred. Here the definition of exposure may be more complex, and it may be necessary to take disease latency periods into account.

Defining Outcomes ("Case Definition")

Establishing a *case definition* is equally important. The case definition is a standard set of criteria for deciding whether an individual should be classified as having the health condition of interest. A case definition includes clinical criteria and, particularly in the setting of an outbreak investigation, restrictions on time, place, and person. The clinical criteria should be simple and objective (e.g., presence of elevated antibody titers, three or more loose bowel movements per day, or illness severe enough to require hospitalization). The case definition may be restricted by time (e.g., to persons with onset of illness within the past 2 months), by place (e.g., to employees of a particular plant or to residents of a metropolitan area), and by person (e.g., to persons with no previous history of pelvic inflammatory disease, or to children at least 9 months old). Whatever the criteria, they must be applied consistently and without bias to all persons under investigation.

COHORT STUDIES

The purpose of a cohort study is to compare the occurrence of disease among two groups of people: those who are exposed and those who are not exposed to a suspected risk factor. This approach permits a direct assessment of the degree of increased risk associated with the exposure.

Thus, cohort studies approximate the paradigm of experimental studies except that the epidemiologist does not determine who is or is not exposed to the risk factor of interest. Some well-known cohort studies have been conducted to study chronic diseases that have long latency periods. In this situation, two groups of people (exposed and unexposed) are monitored for a number of years for the occurrence of disease. A major challenge for such a study is to ensure that follow-up is comparable for both the exposed and unexposed groups.

An alternate approach, and the one used more commonly in field epidemiology, is the "retrospective" cohort study, which relies on historical exposure data. For example, in the typical "church supper" outbreak where all or a representative sample of participants are interviewed, you can compare the rate of disease in those who did or did not eat a certain food—a cohort approach.[3] This retrospective cohort type of study is the technique of choice when one is faced with an acute outbreak in a well-defined population. This method of analysis can also be used in a noninfectious disease context. For example, a cohort of persons exposed to a hazard years ago (e.g., workers exposed to vinyl chloride) is compared to a historically equivalent cohort without this exposure (e.g., workers in a different part of the same plant), and the present vital or disease status in the two groups is compared.[4] This is still a cohort or follow-up study in that the conceptual starting point is exposure status and the risk of disease is compared in the two groups.

However, when the population at risk is not known (e.g., as with nationwide epidemics), the only expedient and scientifically sound way to analyze the problem is to use the case-control method.

ADVANTAGES AND DISADVANTAGES OF COHORT AND CASE-CONTROL STUDY DESIGNS

The relative advantages and disadvantages of the cohort approach mirror the advantages and disadvantages of the case-control approach. These will be compared before case-control studies are discussed in more detail.

Advantages of Cohort Studies/Disadvantages of Case-Control Studies

Risk measurement

One important advantage of the cohort design is that you can directly measure the attack rate or risk of disease. This information is particularly important if the exposure is at the discretion of the individual. Only the cohort study can fill in the blanks of "What is my risk of developing [name of disease] if I choose to [be exposed]?" The case-control approach, which starts with disease status and retrospectively assesses exposure, does not permit a calculation of disease risk for a given exposure group.

Rare exposures

Cohort studies are better suited than case-control studies to examine health effects following a relatively rare exposure. With the cohort approach, all persons with the exposure can be enrolled and followed, as well as a sample of comparable persons who were not exposed. This is the rationale for using the cohort approach in studies of occupational exposures, which are relatively rare in terms of the entire community.

Multiple outcomes

The cohort approach lets you examine the natural history of disease and more than one disease outcome following exposure. Once exposure status is defined, the subjects can be monitored for the occurrence of a variety of disease outcomes. A case-control study, which starts with disease status, does not permit assessment of multiple adverse outcomes associated with exposure.

Potential for bias

To the extent that bias can arise from the definition and selection of comparison groups, cohort studies are less subject to bias than case-control studies. In contrast, questions surrounding the selection of control groups and the resulting potential for bias commonly arise in designing and evaluating case-control studies. This is not to suggest that bias, including confounding bias, cannot occur in cohort studies. For example, if the exposure of interest is defined as residence in a particular community, residents of another community may be defined as the comparison group. If the overall age of members in the two communities differs and if age is associated with the disease in question, then age will confound the comparison of disease risks in the community. In this situation, you would need to adjust for age in the analysis.

Disadvantages of Cohort Studies/Advantages of Case-Control Studies

Logistics/costs

The main disadvantage of a prospective cohort study is its cost and the logistic complexity of following exposed and unexposed persons over time. This problem is heightened if the disease outcome of interest is rare. In this situation, large numbers of exposed and unexposed persons would be required to study the disease outcome and to permit meaningful statistical comparisons. In contrast, case-control studies are relatively inexpensive and are ideally suited to studying rare diseases.

Multiple exposures

Because the starting point in cohort studies is exposure status, it is difficult to examine multiple exposures that may be associated with disease. Because disease status is the starting point in case-control studies, it is possible to question participants retrospectively about a variety of potential exposures.

CASE-CONTROL STUDIES

In a case-control study, people with the disease of interest (cases) are compared to people without the disease. Thus, in defining cases and selecting controls, the cases and controls should be comparable. While this principle appears simple, debates about the selection of controls can be among the most complex in epidemiology.[5] The purpose of this section is to provide an overview and some guidelines. Keep in mind, however, that nearly every generalization about the selection of controls is legitimately arguable.

Objectives of a Case-Control Study

The objective of a case-control study is to measure the association between exposure to a suspected risk factor and disease by comparing exposure among persons who have the disease with exposure among those who do not have the disease.

Purpose of a Control Group

The purpose of the control group is to provide an estimate of exposure (duration, frequency, dose) that would be expected to occur among the case group if there were no association between the exposure and disease.

Criteria for Selection of Controls

The fundamental basis for selecting a control group is that controls should be representative of the population from which the cases arise. In other words, members of this population would be selected as cases for the study (or be eligible for selection) if they had the disease. Suppose your cases have been defined as persons with a particular diagnosis who have been admitted to a single hospital. Your controls should be persons who would be admitted to the same hospital if they had the disease. This is necessary, since persons admitted to a different hospital may reflect different populations (e.g., persons admitted to private hospitals, veterans' hospitals, urban public hospitals, rural hospitals) with a variety of different exposures that may affect the risk of disease. Commonly, controls are selected from the group of patients admitted to the same hospital, but for reasons or diagnoses unrelated to the suspected exposure.

Both cases and controls should have the potential for exposure to the risk factor of interest. Criteria for defining this potential should apply equally to cases and controls.

Suppose that in a preliminary investigation of a suspected food-borne outbreak you have implicated meals served on a particular day at a restaurant. Your initial study of restaurant patrons found a strong association between disease and eating dinner at the restaurant but no association between disease and eating lunch. You then decide to do a second case-control study to identify a particular food item. This second study should be limited to patrons—cases and controls—who ate dinner at the restaurant, excluding patrons who only ate lunch.

Selection of controls (and cases) should be independent of their exposure status. Failure to achieve this independence may bias study results.

Controls should be at risk for the disease. For example, in a study of cigarette smoking and the risk of uterine cancer, it would not be sensible to include men in the control group.

Controls should be free of disease. This underscores the importance of the case definition in distinguishing persons who have the disease from those who do not. For example, if the restaurant-associated outbreak described above were due to an infectious agent, your ability to identify the food source might be reduced if a large number of persons who ate the contaminated food had asymptomatic infections (this would also be a problem for a cohort study). If symptoms alone rather than laboratory results are used to define cases, those asymptomatic infections could be selected as controls. This may reduce the capability of the case-control study to identify an exposure associated with the disease.

For example, in an outbreak of thyrotoxicosis in the mid-1980s, (attributed to eating beef contaminated with thyroid tissue), about 75 percent of asymptomatic family members of patients were found to have elevated thyroid function tests. These asymptomatic family members represent inapparent cases, with the same exposure as the apparent cases. Had they been mistakenly included in the control group, they would have raised the level of exposure among controls and made the exposure-disease association harder to find.[6]

In some situations you can use multiple control groups, and this may overcome the limitations of a single control group. Moreover, if your conclusions are similar when each neighborhood, friend, and hospital control group is compared with cases, then your certainty in interpreting study results would be increased. If the conclusions from analyses of different control groups are inconsistent, then you would have some thinking and explaining to do.

Confounding

Proper selection of controls is one way to protect against bias from confounding in a case-control study. (See also Chapter 8.) Thus, the potential for confounding is an important consideration in selecting a control group.

Confounding can occur when an unstudied risk factor is associated with both the study exposure and the outcome. If confounding is present, the relationship between exposure and disease will be distorted. For example, the risk for many diseases increases with advancing age. If the exposure of interest is more common among older than among younger persons, failure to take age into account in comparing cases and controls will lead to an overestimation of the association between the exposure and disease.

As another example, a case-control study of caffeine consumption and the risk of stroke may produce misleading results if smoking is not considered. This may occur because people who drink coffee are more likely to smoke cigarettes than are people who do not drink coffee and because cigarette smoking is positively associated with the risk of stroke. Here, cigarette smoking (the confounder) is associated with both coffee drinking and the risk of stroke.

Confounding in a case-control study can be reduced by the proper selection of controls or in the analysis. Matching (see below) of controls with cases on the basis of age would eliminate age as a confounder in the above example. Alternatively, age can be taken into account in the analysis by comparing cases and controls separately for different age groups and calculating a weighted, summary measure of the odds ratio (see Chapter 8). Similarly, in the stroke example, cases and controls could be matched for cigarette use, or comparison of coffee drinkers and nondrinkers could later be "stratified" by smoking levels (e.g., nonsmokers, past smokers, or current smokers) in the analysis.

Types of Controls

There are a variety of sources for selecting controls, each with possible strengths and weaknesses in a given situation. Examples include selection among persons served by the same medical care provider, those living in the same area, those who are friends or relatives of cases, or those sampled from the community at large.

In outbreak investigations where a problem has occurred in a well-defined setting, choose the controls from persons in that setting who did not become ill. Examples include well persons who ate at the same meal in a food-borne outbreak or unaffected patients on the same hospital ward in an outbreak of hospital-acquired infection. When an investigation is not limited to a specific location but, for instance, involves the entire United States (e.g., toxic shock syndrome and tampon use, HIV infection and sexual practices, Reye's syndrome and aspirin, female reproductive tract cancers and oral contraceptives), the selection of an appropriate control group is more complex. Options for sources of controls include the following.

Hospital or facility controls

For example, these may include other patients admitted to the same hospital as cases, other patients who are treated by the same physician, or other patients enrolled in the same health maintenance organization. The advantages of this approach are convenience and the assurance that cases and controls are comparable in terms of access to medical care. The disadvantage is that other patients seeking medical care may have conditions that are associated (positively or negatively) with the disease or risk factor of interest. Thus, caution must be taken to avoid selecting control patients whose condition precludes or is related to the study disease or exposure. Selecting patients in different diagnostic categories may offset this hazard.

Friends, relatives, neighbors

Cases may be asked to identify friends, relatives, or neighbors as possible controls. This approach has been useful in the study of rare conditions occurring in geographically diverse areas, and such acquaintances are usually happy to participate in the study. The disadvantage is that friends, relatives, or neighbors may share personal habits and other exposures as the cases. Controls whose exposures are too similar to cases make it harder to identify exposure-disease associations. This situation is called "overmatching."

Community controls

Controls may be randomly selected from the community at large. This method avoids the potential bias in friend controls. Approaches to enlisting controls include door-to-door surveys, mailing, or telephoning. With each approach, however, the inability to reach certain persons may bias study results. For example, telephone surveys would miss persons who do not have telephones, which may or may not be important. In addition, randomly selected community controls are usually less willing to participate in an epidemiologic study.

Sampling Methods for Selecting Controls

A variety of approaches can be used to select controls, depending on the study question, the urgency of an investigation, the resources for the investigation, and the setting.

All persons at risk

In an outbreak with relatively few cases and potential controls, you may select all persons at risk as controls (e.g., all other persons who ate at the suspect meal in a food-borne outbreak, or all other patients admitted to a hospital ward during a nosocomial infections outbreak). In this situation, however, where all affected and unaffected persons are available for study, you have the entire population to study. In this setting, the data should be analyzed in cohort fashion, computing and comparing rates of disease among exposed and unexposed instead of in case-control fashion.

Random or systematic sampling

When you have a roster with a large number of potential controls (e.g., hospital admission records or birth certificates), you can choose a random or systematic sample. For a random sample, you would select persons using a table of random numbers. For a systematic sample, you would select every third or tenth (or other appropriate interval) person on the list.

Pair matching

Matched controls are individually selected on the basis of their similarity to individual cases for certain, predetermined characteristics. Matching criteria are selected because they are potential confounders. Thus, matching on the basis of a particular characteristic eliminates that characteristic as a potential study confounder. Personal characteristics such as age, race/ethnicity, and gender are commonly used as matching criteria when the risk of disease and the likelihood of exposure are both associated with these variables. Matching requires the use of a matched analysis technique.

Matching is advantageous because it is conceptually simple and represents a straightforward way to control for potential confounders. It may be particularly useful in studies where there is a small number of cases available for study.

Matching has some important disadvantages. After selecting matched controls, it is not possible to study the effect of the matching criteria on the study outcome, including interactions between study risk factors and the matching criteria. Matching sometimes requires more effort in finding controls. Matching for variables that are not confounders wastes time and decreases study efficiency.

For example, in an investigation of a nosocomial infection in a newborn intensive care unit, matching by infant birth weight may be done to identify a therapeutic procedure associated with the infection. However, this matching would eliminate the investigators' ability to study birth weight itself as a risk factor.

Frequency matching

Frequency or category matching is an alternative to pair matching. Frequency matching involves selecting controls in proportion to the distribution of certain characteristics of cases. For example, if 75 percent of cases were women, controls would be selected so that 75 percent were women also. This improves the "balance" between cases and controls (and thus study power), so that odds ratios can be determined within strata for matching criteria. As in individual matching, special analytic techniques are required.

In general, pair matching should be avoided unless there is a specific reason for using this approach. Such reasons to use pair matching may include the presence of a small number of cases (which would otherwise render control for confounding difficult in the analysis phase) or the potential for unknown confounders that would be eliminated by matching. In addition, matching may improve the statistical "efficiency" of a study design, permitting the use of a smaller number of cases and controls when a very specific hypothesis is being tested. Alternatives to matching include frequency matching or use of analytic techniques that control for confounding after the data collection (presuming that relevant data can be collected). These include stratified analysis and other multivariate techniques.

Size of Control Group

The number of controls may appropriately be smaller, equal to, or larger than the number of cases, depending on the required level of precision and the number of cases. In matched studies, the matching ratio may be 1:1, 1:2, ctc., or the matching ratio may be variable. In general, little is gained with matching ratios in excess of 1:3 or 1:4.

CONCLUSION

In summary, case-control and cohort studies are the two types of analytic studies used most commonly by epidemiologists in the field. They are effective mechanisms for evaluating—quantifying and testing—hypotheses suggested in earlier phases of the investigation. Cohort studies, which are oriented conceptually from exposure to disease, are appropriate in settings in which the entire population is well defined and available for enrollment (e.g., guests at a wedding reception). Cohort studies are also appropriate when you can define and enroll groups by exposure (e.g., employees working in different parts of a manufacturing plant). More commonly, the population is not as clearly defined, and case-control studies are oriented from disease to exposure: persons with a disease ("cases") are identified through surveillance or other mechanisms, and an appropriate, comparable group of persons without disease ("controls") is selected; then the exposure experiences of the two groups are compared. Though easily said, the specification of an appropriate control group is among the most difficult and judgmental tasks in epidemiology.

REFERENCES

1. Schlesselman, J. J. (1982). *Case-control studies*. Oxford University Press, New York.
2. Rothman, K. J. (1986). *Modern epidemiology*. Little, Brown, Boston.
3. Gross, M. (1976). Oswego County revisited. *Public Health Reports* 91, 160–70.
4. Waxweiler, R. J., Stringer, W., Wagoner, J. K., et al. (1976). Neoplastic risk among workers exposed to vinyl chloride. *Annals of the New York Academy of Sciences* 271, 40–48.
5. Wacholder, S., McLaughlin, J. K., Silverman, D. T., Mandel, J. S. (1992). Selection of controls in case-control studies: I. Principles. *American Journal of Epidemiology* 135, 1019–28.
6. Hedberg, C. W., Fishbein, D. B., Janssen, R. S., et al. (1987). An outbreak of thyrotoxicosis caused by the consumption of bovine thyroid gland in ground beef. *New England Journal of Medicine* 316, 993–98.

8

ANALYZING AND INTERPRETING DATA

Richard C. Dicker

The purpose of many field investigations is to identify causes, risk factors, sources, vehicles, routes of transmission, or other factors that put some members of the population at greater risk than others of having an adverse health event. In some field investigations, identifying a "culprit" is sufficient; if the culprit can be eliminated, the problem is solved. In other field settings, the goal may be to quantify the relationship between exposure (or any population characteristic) and an adverse health event. Quantifying this relationship may lead not only to appropriate interventions but also to advances in knowledge about disease causation. Both types of field investigation require appropriate but not necessarily sophisticated analytic methods. This chapter describes the strategy for planning an analysis, methods for conducting the analysis, and guidelines for interpreting the results.

PREANALYSIS PLANNING

What to Analyze

The first step of a successful analysis is to lay out an analytic strategy in advance. A thoughtfully planned and carefully executed analysis is just as critical for a field investigation as it is for a protocol-based study. Planning is necessary to assure that the appropriate hypotheses will be considered and that the relevant data will be appropriately collected, recorded, managed, analyzed, and interpreted to evaluate those hypotheses. Therefore, the time to decide on what (and how) to analyze the data is before you design your questionnaire, *not* after you have collected the data. As illustrated in Figure 8–1, the hypotheses that you wish to evaluate drive the analysis. (These hypotheses are usually developed by considering the common causes and modes of transmission of the condition under investigation; talking with patients and with local medical and public health staff; observing the dominant patterns in the descriptive epidemiologic data; and scrutinizing the outliers in these data.) Depending on the health condition being investigated, the hypotheses should address the source of the agent, the mode (and vehicle or vector) of transmission, and the exposures that caused disease. They should obviously be testable, since the role of the analysis will be to evaluate them.

Once you have determined the hypotheses to be evaluated, you must decide which data to collect in order to test the hypotheses. (You will also need to determine the best study design to use, as described in the previous chapter.) There is a saying in clinical medicine that "If you don't take a temperature, you can't find a fever".[1] Similarly, in field epidemiology, if you neglect to ask about a potentially important risk factor in the questionnaire, you cannot evaluate its role in the outbreak. Since the hypotheses to be tested dictate the data you need to collect, the time to plan the analysis is before you design the questionnaire.

Questionnaires and other data collection instruments are not limited to risk factors, however. They should also include identifying information, clinical information, and descriptive factors. Identifying information (or ID codes linked to identifying information stored elsewhere) allows you to recontact the respondent to ask additional questions or provide follow-up information. Sufficient clinical information should be collected to determine whether a patient truly meets the case definition. Clinical data on spectrum and severity of illness, hospitalization, and sequelae may also be useful. Descriptive factors related to time, place, and person should be collected to adequately characterize the population, assess comparability between groups (cases and controls in a case-control study; exposed and unexposed groups in a cohort study), and help you generate hypotheses about causal relationships.

Data Editing

Usually, data for an analytic study are collected on paper questionnaires. These data are then entered into a computer. Increasingly, data are entered directly into a computer as they are obtained. In either situation, good data management practices will facilitate the analysis. These practices include, at the very least,

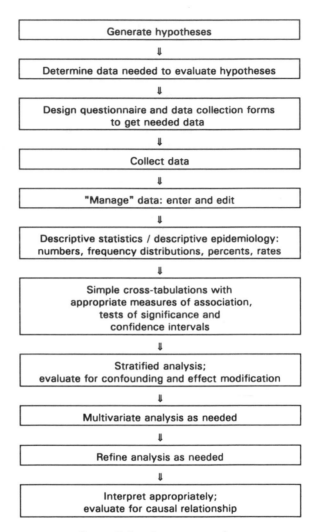

Figure 8–1.   Steps in an analysis.

- Ensuring that you have the right number of records, with no duplicates
- Performing quality-control checks on each data field

Check that the number of records in the computerized database matches the number of questionnaires. Then check for duplicate records. It is not uncommon for questionnaires to be skipped or entered twice, particularly if they are not all entered at one sitting.

Two types of quality-control checks should be performed before beginning the analysis: range checks and logic (or consistency) checks. A range check identifies values for each variable that are "out of range" (i.e., not allowed, or at least highly suspicious). If, for the variable "gender," "male" is coded as 1 and "female" as 2, the range check should flag all records with any value other than 1 or 2. If 3's, F's, or blanks are found, review the original questionnaire, recontact the respondent, or recode those values to "known missing." For the variable "weight (in pounds)," an allowable range for adults might be 90 to 250. It is quite possible that some respondents will weigh more or less than this range, but it is also possible that values outside that range represent coding errors. Again, you must decide whether to attempt to verify the information or leave it as entered. The effort needed to confirm and complete the information should be weighed against the effect of lost data in the analysis—for a small study, you can ill afford missing data for the key variables but can tolerate it for less important variables. Under no circumstances should you change a value just because "it doesn't seem right."

A logic check compares responses to two different questions and flags those that are inconsistent. For example, a record in which "gender" is coded as "male" and "hysterectomy" is coded as "yes" should probably be flagged! Dates can also be compared—date of onset of illness should usually precede date of hospitalization (except in outbreaks of nosocomial infection, when date of hospitalization *precedes* date of onset) and date of onset should precede date of report. Again you must decide how to handle inconsistencies.

Two additional principles should guide data management. First, document everything, particularly your decisions. Take a blank copy of the questionnaire and write the name of each variable next to the corresponding question on the questionnaire. If, for the variable "gender," you decide to recode F's as 2's and recode 3's and blanks as 9's for "known missing," write those decisions down as well, so that you and others will know how to recode unacceptable values for gender in the future.

Note that you cannot create logic checks in advance for every possible contingency. Many inconsistencies in a database come to light during the analysis. Treat these inconsistencies the same way—decide how best to resolve the inconsistency (short of making up better data!) and then document your decision.

The second principle is, "Never let an error age." Deal with the problem as soon as you find it. Under the pressures of a field investigation, it is all too common to forget about a data error, analyze the data as they are, and then be embarrassed during a presentation when calculations or values in a table do not seem to make sense.

Developing the Analysis Strategy

After the data have been edited, they are ready to be analyzed. But before you sit down to analyze the data, first develop an analysis strategy (Table 8–1). The analysis

Table 8–1. Sequence of an Epidemiologic Analysis Strategy

---

1. Establish how the data were collected and plan to analyze accordingly.
2. Identify and list the most important variables in light of what you know about the subject matter, biologically plausible hypotheses, and the manner in which the study will be (or was) conducted:
   Exposures of interest
   Outcomes of interest
   Potential confounders
   Variables for subgroup analysis
3. To become familiar with the data, plan to perform frequency distributions and descriptive statistics on the variables identified in step 2.
4. To characterize the study population, create tables of clinical features and descriptive epidemiology (table shells should be created in advance).
5. To assess exposure-disease associations, create two-way tables based on study design, prior knowledge, and hypotheses (table shells should be created in advance).
6. Create additional two-way tables based on interesting findings in the data.
7. Create three-way tables, refinements (e.g., dose-response; sensitivity analysis) and subgroup analysis based on design, prior knowledge, hypotheses, or interesting findings in the data.

---

strategy is comparable to the outline you would develop before sitting down to write a term paper. It lays out the key components of the analysis in a logical sequence and provides a guide to follow during the actual analysis. An analytic strategy that is well planned in advance will expedite the analysis once the data are collected.

The first step in developing the analysis strategy is recognizing how the data were collected. For example, if you have data from a cohort study, think in terms of exposure groups and plan to calculate rates. If you have data from a case-control study, think in terms of cases and controls. If the cases and controls were matched, plan to do a matched analysis. If you have survey data, review the sampling scheme— you may need to account for the survey's design effect in your analysis.

The next step is deciding which variables are most important. Include the exposures and outcomes of interest, other known risk factors, study design factors such as variables you matched on, any other variables you think may have an impact on the analysis, and variables you are simply interested in. In a small questionnaire, perhaps all variables will be deemed important. Plan to review the frequency of responses and descriptive statistics for each variable. This is the best way to become familiar with the data. What are the minimum, maximum, and average values for each variable? Are there any variables that have many missing responses? If you hope to do a stratified or subgroup analysis by, say, race, is there a sufficient number of responses in each race category?

The next step in the analysis strategy is sketching out table shells. A table shell (sometimes called a "dummy table") is a table such as a frequency distribution or two-way table that is titled and fully labeled but contains no data. The numbers will be filled in as the analysis progresses.

You should sketch out the series of table shells as a guide for the analysis. The table shells should proceed in a logical order from simple (e.g., descriptive epidemiology) to complex (e.g., analytic epidemiology). The table shells should also indicate which measures (e.g., odds ratio) and statistics (e.g., chi square) you will calculate for each table. Measures and statistics are described later in this chapter.

One way to think about the types and sequence of table shells is to consider what tables you would want to show in a report. One common sequence is as follows:

Table 1: Clinical features (e.g., signs and symptoms, percent lab-confirmed, percent hospitalized, percent died, etc.)
Table 2: Descriptive epidemiology
Time: usually graphed as line graph (for secular trends) or epidemic curve
Place: (county of residence or occurrence, spot or shaded map)
Person: "Who is in the study?" (age, race, gender, etc.)

For analytic studies,

Table 3: Primary tables of association (i.e., risk factors by outcome status)
Table 4: Stratification of Table 3 to separate effects and to assess confounding and effect modification
Table 5: Refinements of Table 3 (e.g., dose-response, latency, use of more sensitive or more specific case definition, etc.)
Table 6: Specific subgroup analyses

The following sequence of table shells (A through I) was designed before conducting a case-control study of Kawasaki syndrome (a pediatric disease of unknown cause that occasionally occurs in clusters). Since there is no definitive diagnostic test for this syndrome, the case definition requires that the patient have fever plus at least four of five other clinical findings listed in Table Shell A. Three hypotheses to be tested by the case-control study were the syndrome's purported association with antecedent viral illness, recent exposure to carpet shampoo, and increasing household income.

Since descriptive epidemiology has been covered in Chapter 5, the remainder of this chapter addresses the analytic techniques most commonly used in field investigations.

Table Shell A. Diagnostic Criteria for Kawasaki Syndrome Cases
with Onset October–December

CRITERION	NUMBER	PERCENT
1. Fever ≥ 5 days	—	(%)
2. Bilateral conjunctival injection	—	(%)
3. Oral changes	—	(%)
Injected lips	—	(%)
Injected pharynx	—	(%)
Dry, fissured lips	—	(%)
Strawberry tongue	—	(%)
4. Peripheral extremity changes	—	(%)
Edema	—	(%)
Erythema	—	(%)
Periungual desquamation	—	(%)
5. Rash	—	(%)
6. Cervical lymphadenopathy > 1.5 cm	—	(%)

Table Shell B. Days of Hospitalization, Kawasaki Syndrome Cases
with Onset October–December

DAYS OF HOSPITALIZATION	FREQUENCY
0	—
1	—
2	—
3	—
4	—
5	—
6	—
7	—
8	—
9	—
and so on to maximum	—
Unknown	—
Range:	—
Mean:	—
Median:	—

Table Shell C. Frequency Distribution of Serious Complications among Kawasaki Syndrome Cases with Onset October–December

CRITERION	NUMBER	PERCENT
Arthritis	—	(%)
Coronary artery aneurysm	—	(%)
Other complications (list:)	—	(%)
Death	—	(%)

Table Shell D. Demographic Characteristics of Kawasaki Syndrome Cases with Onset October–December

DEMOGRAPHIC CHARACTERISTIC		NUMBER	PERCENT
Age	< 1 yr	—	(%)
	1 yr	—	(%)
	2 yr	—	(%)
	3 yr	—	(%)
	4 yr	—	(%)
	5 yr	—	(%)
	≥ 6 yr	—	(%)
Gender	Male	—	(%)
	Female	—	(%)
Race	White	—	(%)
	Black	—	(%)
	Asian	—	(%)
	Other	—	(%)

Table Shell E. Frequency Distribution by County of Residence, Kawasaki Syndrome Cases, October–December

COUNTY	NUMBER	PERCENT	POPULATION	ATTACK RATE
County A	—	(%)	—	—
County B	—	(%)	—	—
County C	—	(%)	—	—
County D	—	(%)	—	—
County E	—	(%)	—	—
County F	—	(%)	—	—

Table Shell F. Frequency Distribution by Household Income,
Kawasaki Syndrome Cases, October–December

ANNUAL HOUSEHOLD INCOME[a]	NUMBER	PERCENT
< $15,000	—	(%)
$15,000–$29,999	—	(%)
$30,000–$44,999	—	(%)
≥ $45,000	—	(%)

[a]May need to revise categories of household income to portray range.

Table Shell G. Kawasaki Syndrome and Antecedent Illness, Case Control Study

		CASES	CONTROLS	TOTAL	
ANTECEDENT ILLNESS	YES	—	—	—	Odds ratio = ___ 95% CI = (,)
	NO	—	—	—	x^2 = _____ , P value = _____
	TOTAL	—	—		

Table Shell H. Kawasaki Syndrome and Carpet Shampoo, Case Control Study

		CASES	CONTROLS	TOTAL	
CARPET SHAMPOO	YES	—	—	—	Odds ratio = ___ 95% CI = (,)
	NO	—	—	—	x^2 = _____ , P value = _____
	TOTAL	—	—	—	

Table Shell I. Kawasaki Syndrome and Carpet Shampoo, Case Control Study

		CASES	CONTROLS	TOTAL	
HOUSEHOLD INCOME (IN THOUSANDS OF DOLLARS)	<15	—	—	—	
	15–30	—	—	—	x^2 = _____ ,
	30–45	—	—	—	P value = _____
	45+	—	—	—	
	TOTAL	—	—	—	

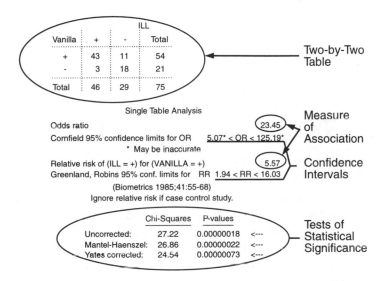

Figure 8–2. Typical *Epi Info* output from the analysis module, using the "tables" command. *Source:* CDC (1994).

Figure 8–2 depicts a screen from *Epi Info*'s Analysis module (see Chapter 12). It shows the output from the "Tables" command for data from a typical field investigation. Note the four elements of the output: (1) a two-by-two table, (2) measures of association, (3) tests of statistical significance, and (4) confidence intervals. Each of these elements is discussed below.

The Two-by-Two Table

"Every epidemiologic study can be summarized in a two-by-two table."

—H. Ory

In many epidemiologic studies, exposure and the health event being studied can be characterized as binary variables (e.g., "yes" or "no"). The relationship between exposure and disease can then be cross-tabulated in a *two-by-two table*, so named because both the exposure and disease have just two categories (Table 8–2). One can put disease status (e.g., ill vs. well) along the top and exposure status along the side. (*Epi Info*, a microcomputer program written for field use, also follows this convention, although some epidemiologic textbooks do not [see Chapter 12].) The intersection of a row and a column in which a count is recorded is known as a *cell*. The letters a, b, c, and d within the four cells of the two-by-two table refer to the number of persons with the disease status indicated in the column heading and the exposure status indicated to the left. For example, c is the number of unexposed ill/case subjects in the study. The *horizontal* row totals are labeled h_1

Table 8–2. Data layout and notation for standard two-by-two table.

	ILL	WELL	TOTAL	ATTACK RATE
EXPOSED	a	b	h_1	a/h_1
UNEXPOSED	c	d	h_0	c/h_0
TOTAL	v_1	v_0	t	v_1/t

and h_0 (or h_2), and the *vertical* column totals are labeled v_1 and v_0 (or v_2). The total number of subjects included in the two-by-two table is written in the lower right corner and is represented by the letter t or n. Attack rates (the proportion of a group of people who develop disease during a specified time interval) are sometimes provided to the right of the row totals.

Data from an outbreak investigation in South Carolina are presented in Table 8–3. The table provides a cross-tabulation of turkey consumption (exposure) by presence or absence of *Salmonella* gastroenteritis (outcome). Attack rates (56.4 percent for those who ate turkey; 12.2 percent for those who did not) are given to the right of the table.

MEASURES OF ASSOCIATION

A measure of association quantifies the strength or magnitude of the statistical association between the exposure and the health problem of interest. Measures of association are sometimes called measures of effect because—if the exposure is causally related to the disease—the measures quantify the effect of having the exposure on the incidence of disease. In cohort studies, the measure of association most commonly used is the relative risk. In case-control studies, the odds ratio is the most commonly used measure of association. In cross-sectional studies, either a prevalence ratio or a prevalence odds ratio may be calculated.

Table 8–3. Turkey Consumption and Gastrointestinal Illness, *Salmonella* Outbreak, South Carolina, 1990

		ILL	WELL	TOTAL	ATTACK RATE
ATE	YES	115	89	204	56.4%
TURKEY?	NO	5	36	41	12.2%
	TOTAL	120	125	245	49.0%

Source: Luby et al. (1993).[2]

Relative Risk (Risk Ratio)

The relative risk is the risk in the exposed group divided by the risk in the unexposed group:

$$\text{Relative risk (RR)} = \text{risk}_{\text{exposed}} / \text{risk}_{\text{unexposed}} = (a/h_1) / (c/h_0)$$

The relative risk reflects the excess risk in the exposed group compared with the unexposed (background, expected) group. The excess is expressed as a ratio. In acute outbreak settings, risk is represented by the attack rate. The data presented in Table 8–3 show that the relative risk of illness, given turkey consumption, was $0.564/0.122 = 4.6$. That is, persons who ate turkey were 4.6 times more likely to become ill than those who did not eat turkey. Note that the relative risk will be greater than 1.0 when the risk is greater in the exposed group than in the unexposed group. The relative risk will be less than 1.0 when the risk in the exposed group is less than the risk in the unexposed group, as is usually the case when the exposure under study is vaccination.

Odds Ratio (Cross-Product Ratio, Relative Odds)

In most case-control studies, because you do not know the true size of the exposed and unexposed groups, you do not have a denominator with which to calculate an attack rate or risk. However, using case control data, the relative risk can be approximated by an odds ratio. The odds ratio is calculated as

$$\text{Odds ratio (OR)} = ad/bc$$

In an outbreak of group A *Streptococcus* (GAS) surgical wound infections in a community hospital, 10 cases had occurred during a 17-month period. Investigators used a table of random numbers to select controls from the 2,600 surgical procedures performed during the epidemic period. Since many clusters of GAS surgical wound infections can be traced to a GAS carrier among operating room

Table 8–4. Surgical Wound Infection and Exposure to Nurse A, Hospital M, Michigan, 1980

		CASE	CONTROL	TOTAL
EXPOSED TO	YES	8	5	13
NURSE A?	NO	2	49	51
	TOTAL	10	54	64

Source: Berkelman et al. (1982).[3]

personnel, investigators studied all hospital staff associated with each patient. They drew a two-by-two table for exposure to each staff member and calculated odds ratios. The two-by-two table for exposure to nurse A is shown in Table 8–4. The odds ratio is calculated as $8 \times 49/2 \times 5 = 39.2$. Strictly speaking, this means that the *odds* of being exposed to nurse A were 39 times higher among cases than among controls. It is also reasonable to say that the odds of developing a GAS surgical wound infection were 39 times higher among those exposed to nurse A than among those not exposed. For a rare disease (say, less than 5 percent), the odds ratio approximates the relative risk. So in this setting, with only 10 cases out of 2,600 procedures, the odds ratio could be interpreted as indicating that the *risk* of developing a GAS surgical wound infection was 39 times higher among those exposed to nurse A than among those not exposed.

The odds ratio is a very useful measure of association in epidemiology for a variety of reasons. As noted above, when the disease is rare, a case-control study can yield an odds ratio that closely approximates the relative risk from a cohort study. From a theoretical statistical perspective (beyond the scope of this book), the odds ratio also has some desirable statistical properties and is easily derived from multivariate modeling techniques.

Prevalence Ratio and Prevalence Odds Ratio

Cross-sectional studies or surveys generally measure the prevalence (existing cases) of a health condition in a population rather than the incidence (new cases). Prevalence is a function of both incidence (risk) and duration of illness, so measures of association based on prevalent cases reflect both the exposure's effect on incidence and its effect on duration or survival.

The prevalence measures of association analogous to the relative risk and the odds ratio are the *prevalence ratio* and the *prevalence odds* ratio, respectively.

In the two-by-two table (Table 8–5), the prevalence ratio = 0.20/0.05 = 4.0. That is, exposed subjects are four times as likely as are unexposed subjects to have the condition. In the example above, the prevalence odds ratio = (20) (380) / (80) (20) = 4.75. The *odds* of having disease is 4.75 times higher for the exposed than the unexposed group. Note that when the prevalence is low, the values of the prevalence ratio and the prevalence odds ratio will be similar.

MEASURES OF PUBLIC HEALTH IMPACT

A measure of public health impact places the exposure-disease association in a public health perspective. It reflects the apparent contribution of an exposure to the frequency of disease in a particular population. For example, for an exposure

Table 8–5. Data from a Hypothetical Cross-Sectional Survey

		HAVE CONDITION?			
		YES	NO	TOTAL	PREVALENCE
EXPOSED?	YES	20	80	100	0.20
	NO	20	380	400	0.05
	TOTAL	40	460	500	

associated with an increased risk of disease (e.g., smoking and lung cancer), the attributable risk percent represents the expected reduction in disease load if the exposure could be removed (or never existed). The population attributable risk percent represents the proportion of disease in a population attributable to an exposure. For an exposure associated with a decreased risk of disease (e.g., vaccination), a prevented fraction could be calculated that represents the actual reduction in disease load attributable to the current level of exposure in the population.

Attributable Risk Percent (Attributable Fraction [or Proportion] among the Exposed, Etiologic Fraction)

The attributable risk percent is the proportion of cases in the exposed group presumably attributable to the exposure. This measure assumes that the level of risk in the unexposed group (assumed to be the baseline or background risk of disease) also applies to the exposed group, so that only the *excess* risk should be attributed to the exposure. The attributable risk percent can be calculated with either of the following formulas (which are algebraically equivalent):

$$\text{Attributable risk percent} = (\text{risk}_{\text{exposed}} - \text{risk}_{\text{unexposed}}) / \text{risk}_{\text{exposed}}$$
$$= (RR - 1) / RR$$

The attributable risk percent can be reported as a fraction or can be multiplied by 100 and reported as a percent. Using the turkey consumption data in Table 8–3, the attributable risk percent is $(0.564 - 0.122) / 0.564 = 78.4$ percent. Therefore, over three-fourths of the gastroenteritis that occurred among persons who ate turkey may be attributable to turkey consumption. The other 21.6 percent is attributed to the baseline occurrence of gastroenteritis in that population.

In a case-control study, if the odds ratio is thought to be a reasonable approximation of the relative risk, you can calculate the attributable risk percent as

$$\text{Attributable risk percent} = (OR - 1) / OR$$

Population Attributable Risk Percent (Population Attributable Fraction)

The population attributable risk percent is the proportion of cases in the entire population (both exposed and unexposed groups) presumably attributable to the exposure. Algebraically equivalent formulas include

$$\text{Population attributable risk percent} = (\text{risk}_{overall} - \text{risk}_{unexposed}) / \text{risk}_{overall}$$
$$= P(RR - 1) / [P(RR - 1) + 1]$$

where P = proportion of population exposed = h_1/t

Applying the first formula to the turkey consumption data, the population attributable risk percent is $(0.490 - 0.122) / 0.490 = 75.1$ percent. In situations in which most of the cases are exposed, the attributable risk percent and population attributable risk percent will be close. For diseases with multiple causes (e.g., many chronic diseases) and uncommon exposures, the population attributable risk percent may be considerably less than the attributable risk percent.

The population attributable risk percent can be estimated from a population-based case-control study by using the OR to approximate the RR and by using the proportion of controls exposed to approximate P; that is, $P = b/v_0$ (assuming that the controls are representative of the entire population).

Prevented Fraction in the Exposed Group (Vaccine Efficacy)

If the risk ratio is less than 1.0, you can calculate the prevented fraction, which is the proportion of potential new cases that would have occurred in the absence of the exposure. In other words, the prevented fraction is the proportion of potential cases prevented by some beneficial exposure, such as vaccination. The prevented fraction in the exposed group is calculated as

$$\text{Prevented fraction among the exposed} = (\text{risk}_{unexposed} - \text{risk}_{exposed}) / \text{risk}_{unexposed}$$
$$= 1 - RR$$

Table 8–5 presents data from a 1970 measles outbreak along the Texas-Arkansas border. Because some cases had occurred among children vaccinated against measles, the public questioned the effectiveness of the measles vaccine. As shown in Table 8–6, the risk of measles among vaccinated children was about 4 percent of the risk among unvaccinated children. Vaccine efficacy was calculated to be 96 percent indicating that vaccination prevented 96 percent of the cases that might have otherwise occurred among vaccinated children had they not been vaccinated.

Table 8–6. Vaccination Status and Occurrence of Measles, Texarkana, 1970

	MEASLES	NO MEASLES	TOTAL	RISK PER 1,000	RELATIVE RISK
VACCINATED	27	6,323	6,350	4.2	0.04
NOT VACCINATED	512	4,323	4,835	105.9	(REFERENCE)
TOTAL	539	10,646	11,185	48.2	

Vaccine efficacy = (105.9 – 4.2) / 105.9 = 0.96

Source: Landrigan (1972).[4]

Note that the terms "attributable" and "prevented" convey much more than statistical association. They imply a cause-and-effect relationship between the exposure and disease. Therefore, these measures should not be presented routinely but only after thoughtful inference of causality.

TESTS OF STATISTICAL SIGNIFICANCE

Tests of statistical significance are used to determine how likely it is that the observed results could have occurred by chance alone, if exposure was not actually related to disease. In the paragraphs below, we describe the key features of the tests most commonly used with two-by-two tables. For discussion of theory, derivations, and other topics beyond the scope of this book, we suggest that you consult one of the many biostatistics textbooks, which cover these subjects well.

In statistical testing, you assume that the study population is a sample from some large "source population." Then assume that, in the source population, incidence of disease is the same for exposed and unexposed groups. In other words, assume that, in the source population, exposure is not related to disease. This assumption is known as the *null hypothesis*. (The *alternative hypothesis*, which may be adopted if the null hypothesis proves to be implausible, is that exposure *is* associated with disease.) Next, compute a measure of association, such as a relative risk or odds ratio. Then, calculate the test of statistical significance such as a chi square (described below). This test tells you the probability of finding an association as strong as (or stronger than) the one you have observed if the null hypothesis were really true. This probability is called the *P value*. A very small *P* value means that you would be very unlikely to observe such an association if the null hypothesis were true. In other words, a small *P* value indicates that the null hypothesis is implausible, given the data at hand. If this *P* value is smaller than some predetermined cutoff (usually 0.05 or 5 percent), you can discard ("reject") the null hypothesis in favor of the alternative hypothesis.The association is then said to be "statistically significant."

In reaching a decision about the null hypothesis, be alert to two types of error. In a *type I error* (also called *alpha error*), the null hypothesis is rejected when in fact it is true. In a *type II error* (also called *beta error*), the null hypothesis is not rejected when in fact it is false.

Both the null hypothesis and the alternative hypothesis should be specified in advance. When little is known about the association being tested, you should specify a null hypothesis that the exposure is not related to disease (e.g., $RR = 1$ or $OR = 1$). The corresponding alternative hypothesis states that exposure and disease are associated (e.g., $RR \neq 1$ or $OR \neq 1$). Note that this alternative hypothesis includes the possibilities that exposure may either increase or decrease the risk of disease.

When you know more about the association between a given exposure and disease, you may specify a narrower ("directional") hypothesis. For example, if it is well established that an exposure increases the risk of developing a particular health problem (e.g., smoking and lung cancer), you can specify a null hypothesis that the exposure does not increase risk of that condition (e.g., $RR \leq 1$ or $OR \leq 1$) and an alternative hypothesis that exposure does increase the risk (e.g., $RR > 1$ or $OR > 1$). Similarly, if you were studying a well-established protective relationship [measles-mumps-rubella (MMR) vaccine and measles], you could specify a null hypothesis that $RR \geq 1$ and an alternative hypothesis that $RR < 1$.

A nondirectional hypothesis is tested by a "two-tailed" test. A directional hypothesis is tested with a "one-tailed" test. In general, the cutoff for a one-tailed test is twice the cutoff of a two-tailed test (i.e., 0.10 rather than 0.05). Since raising the cutoff for rejecting the null hypothesis increases the likelihood of making a type I error, epidemiologists in field situations generally use a two-tailed test.

Two different tests, each with some variations, are used for testing data in a two-by-two table. These two tests, described below, are the Fisher exact test and the chi-square test. These tests are not specific to any particular measure of association. The same test can be used regardless of whether you are interested in risk ratio, odds ratio, or attributable risk.

Fisher Exact Test

The Fisher exact test is considered the "gold standard" for a two-by-two table and is the test of choice when the numbers in a two-by-two table are small. Assume that the null hypothesis is true in the source population and that the values in the four cells but not the row and column totals of the two-by-two table could change. The Fisher exact test involves computing the probability of observing an association in a sample equal to or greater than the one observed. The technique for deriving this probability is outlined in Appendix 8–1.

As a rule of thumb, the Fisher exact test is the test of choice when the *expected* value in any cell of the two-by-two table is less than 5. The expected value is calculated by multiplying the row total by the column total and dividing by the table total. However, calculating the Fisher exact test, which is tedious at best for small numbers, becomes virtually impossible when the numbers get large. Fortunately, with large numbers, the chi-square test provides a reasonable approximation to the Fisher exact test.

Chi-Square Test

When you have at least 30 subjects and the expected value in each cell of the two-by-two table is at least 5, the chi-square test provides a reasonable approximation to the Fisher exact test. Plugging the appropriate numbers into the chi-square formula, you get a value for the Chi-square. Then look up its corresponding two-tailed *P* value in a chi-square table (see Appendix 8–2). A two-by-two table has one degree of freedom,* and a chi-square larger than 3.84 corresponds to a two-tailed *P* value smaller than 0.05.

At least three different formulas of the chi-square for a two-by-two table are in common use; *Epi Info* presents all three.

$$\text{Pearson uncorrected } \chi^2 = \frac{t\,(ad-bc)^2}{(v_1)\,(v_0)\,(h_1)\,(h_0)}$$

$$\text{Yates corrected } \chi^2 = \frac{t\,\left(\left|ad-bc\right| - \left(\frac{t}{2}\right)\right)^2}{(v_1)\,(v_0)\,(h_1)\,(h_0)}$$

$$\text{Mantel-Haenzel } \chi^2 = \frac{(t-1)\,(ad-bc)^2}{(v_1)\,(v_0)\,(h_1)\,(h_0)}$$

For a given set of data in a two-by-two table, the Pearson chi-square formula gives the largest chi-square value and hence the smallest *P* value. This *P* value is often somewhat smaller than the "gold standard" *P* value calculated by the Fisher exact method. So the Pearson chi-square is more apt to lead to a type I error (concluding that there is an association when there is not). The Yates corrected chi square gives the largest *P* value of the three formulas, sometimes even larger than the corresponding Fisher exact *P* value. The Yates correction is preferred by those epidemiologists who want to minimize their likelihood of making a type I error, but it increases the likelihood of making a type II error. The Mantel-Haenszel formula, popular in stratified analysis,

---

*Degrees of freedom equals the number of rows in the table minus 1 times the number of columns in the table minus 1. So for a two-by-two table, degrees of freedom = $(2 - 1) \times (2 - 1) = 1$.

yields a P value which is slightly larger than that from the Pearson chi square but often smaller than the P value from the Yates corrected chi square and Fisher exact P value. Table 8–7 shows the data for macaroni consumption and risk of gastroenteritis from the South Carolina *Salmonella* outbreak. For these data, the Pearson and Mantel-Haenszel chi-square formulas yield P values smaller than 0.05 (the usual cutoff for rejecting the null hypothesis). In contrast, the corrected chi-square formula yields a P value closer to but slightly larger than the Fisher exact P value (the "gold standard"). Both P values are larger than 0.05, indicating that the null hypothesis should *not* be rejected. Fortunately, for most analyses the three chi-square formulas provide similar enough P values to make the same decision regarding the null hypothesis based on all three.

Which Test to Use?

The Fisher exact test should be used if the expected value in any cell is less than 5. Remember that the expected value for any cell can be determined by multiplying the row total by the column total and dividing by the table total.

Table 8–7. Macaroni Consumption and Gastroenteritis, *Salmonella* Outbreak, South Carolina, 1990

	ILL	WELL	TOTAL	RISK	
EXPOSED	76	63	139	54.7%	Relative risk = 1.3
UNEXPOSED	44	62	106	41.5%	Odds ratio = 1.7
TOTAL	120	125	245		

$$\text{Uncorrected } \chi^2 = \frac{(245)\,(76 \times 62 - 63 \times 44)^2}{(120)\,(125)\,(139)\,(106)} = 4.17$$

$$\text{Mantel-Haenszel } \chi^2 = \frac{(245 - 1)\,(76 \times 62 - 63 \times 44)^2}{(120)\,(125)\,(139)\,(106)} = 4.16$$

$$\text{Corrected } \chi^2 = \frac{(245)\,[|76 \times 62 - 63 \times 44| - (\frac{245}{2})]^2}{(120)\,(125)\,(139)\,(106)} = 3.66$$

The corresponding two-tailed P values are as follows:

Uncorrected $\chi^2 = 4.17$, P value = 0.041
Mantel-Haenszel $\chi^2 = 4.16$, P value = 0.042
Corrected $\chi^2 = 3.66$, P value = 0.056

Fisher exact P value (two-tail) = 0.053

Source: Luby et al. (1993).[2]

If all expected values in the two-by-two table are 5 or greater, then you can choose among the chi-square tests. Each of the three formulas shown above has its advocates among epidemiologists, and *Epi Info* provides all three. Many field epidemiologists prefer the Yates corrected formula because they are least likely to make type I error (but most likely to make a type II error). Epidemiologists who frequently perform stratified analyses are accustomed to using the Mantel-Haenszel formula, so they tend to use this formula even for simple two-by-two tables.

Measure of Association versus Test of Significance

The measures of association, such as relative risk and odds ratio, reflect the strength of the relationship between an exposure and a disease. These measures are generally independent of the size of the study and may be thought of as the "best guess" of the true degree of association in the source population. However, the measure gives no indication of its reliability (i.e., how much faith to put in it).

In contrast, a test of significance provides an indication of how likely it is that the observed association may be due to chance. Although the chi-square test statistic is influenced both by the magnitude of the association and the study size, it does not distinguish the contribution of each one. Thus the measure of association and the test of significance (or a confidence interval, see below) provide complementary information.

Interpreting Statistical Test Results

"Not significant" does not necessarily mean "no association." The measure of association (relative risk, odds ratio) indicates the direction and strength of the association. The statistical test indicates how likely it is that the observed association may have occurred by chance alone. Nonsignificance may reflect no association in the source population but may also reflect a study size too small to detect a true association in the source population.

Statistical significance does not by itself indicate a cause-effect relationship. An observed association may indeed represent a causal relationship, but it may also be due to chance, selection bias, information bias, confounding, and other sources of error in the design, execution, and analysis of the study. Statistical testing relates only to the role of chance in explaining an observed association, and statistical significance indicates only that chance is an unlikely (though not impossible) explanation of the association. You must rely on your epidemiologic judgment in considering these factors as well as consistency of the findings with those from other studies, the temporal relationship between exposure and disease, biological plausibility, and other criteria for inferring causation. These issues are discussed at greater length in the last section of this chapter.

Finally, statistical significance does not necessarily mean public health significance. With a large study, a weak association with little public health (or clinical) relevance many nonetheless be "statistically significant." More commonly, relationships of public health and/or clinical importance fail to be "statistically significant" because the studies are too small.

CONFIDENCE INTERVALS FOR MEASURES OF ASSOCIATION

We have just described the use of a statistical test to determine how likely the difference between an observed association and the null state is consistent with chance variation. Another index of the statistical variability of the association is the *confidence interval*. Statisticians define a 95% confidence interval as the interval that, given repeated sampling of the source population, will include or "cover" the true association value 95 percent of the time. The confidence interval from a single study may be roughly interpreted as the range of values that, given the data at hand and in the absence of bias, has a 95 percent chance of including the "true" value. Even more loosely, the confidence interval may be thought of as the range in which the "true" value of an association is likely to be found, or the range of values that is consistent with the data in your study.

The chi-square test and the confidence interval are closely related. The chi-square test uses the observed data to determine the probability (*P* value) under the null hypothesis, and you "reject" the null hypothesis if the probability is less than some preselected value, called alpha, such as 5 percent. The confidence interval uses a preselected probability value, alpha, to determine the limits of the interval, and you can reject the null hypothesis if the interval does not include the null association value. Both indicate the precision of the observed association; both are influenced by the magnitude of the association and the size of the study group. While both measure precision, neither addresses validity (lack of bias).

You must select a probability level (alpha) to determine limiting values of the confidence interval. As with the chi-square test, epidemiologists traditionally choose an alpha level of 0.05 or 0.01. The "confidence" is then 100 x (1 − alpha) percent (e.g., 95 percent or 99 percent).

Unlike the calculation of a chi square, the calculation of a confidence interval is a function of the particular measure of association. That is, each association measure has its own formula for calculating confidence intervals. In fact, each measure has several formulas. There are "exact" confidence intervals and a variety of approximations.

Interpreting the Confidence Interval

As noted above, a confidence interval is sometimes loosely regarded as the range of values consistent with the data in a study. Suppose that you conducted a study in your area in which the relative risk for smoking and disease X was 4.0, and the 95 percent confidence interval was 3.0 to 5.3. Your single best guess of the association in the general population is 4.0, but your data are consistent with values anywhere from 3.0 to 5.3. Note that your data are *not* consistent with a relative risk of 1.0; that is, your data are *not* consistent with the null hypothesis. Thus, the values that are included in the confidence interval and values that are excluded both provide important information.

The width of a confidence interval (i.e., the values included) reflects the precision with which a study can pinpoint an association such as a relative risk. A wide confidence interval reflects a large amount of variability or imprecision. A narrow confidence interval reflects little variability and high precision. Usually, the larger the number of subjects or observations in a study, the greater the precision and the narrower the confidence interval.

As stated earlier, the measure of association provides the "best guess" of our estimate of the true association. If we were in a casino, that "best guess" would be the number to bet on. The confidence interval provides a measure of the confidence we should have in that "best guess," that is, it tells us how much to bet! A wide confidence interval indicates a fair amount of imprecision in our best guess, so we should not bet too much on that one number. A narrow confidence interval indicates a more precise estimate, so we might want to bet more on that number.

Since a confidence interval reflects the range of values consistent with the data in a study, one can use the confidence interval to determine whether the data are consistent with the null hypothesis. Since the null hypothesis specifies that the relative risk (or odds ratio) equals 1.0, a confidence interval that includes 1.0 is consistent with the null hypothesis. This is equivalent to deciding that the null hypothesis cannot be rejected. On the other hand, a confidence interval that does not include 1.0 indicates that the null hypothesis should be rejected, since it is inconsistent with the study results. Thus the confidence interval can be used as a test of statistical significance.

SUMMARY EXPOSURE TABLES

If the goal of the field investigation is to identify one or more vehicles or risk factors for disease, it may be helpful to summarize the exposures of interest in a single table, such as Table 8–8. For a food-borne outbreak, the table typically includes each food item served, numbers of ill and well persons by food consumption history, food-specific attack rates (if a cohort study was done), relative risk (or odds ratio), chi square and/or P value, and, sometimes, a confidence interval. To identify a culprit, you should look for a food item with two features:

1. An elevated relative risk, odds ratio, or chi square (small P value), reflecting a substantial difference in attack rates among those exposed to the item and those not exposed.
2. Most of the ill persons had been exposed, so that the exposure could "explain" most if not all of the cases.

In Table 8–8, turkey has the highest relative risk (and smallest P value) and can account for 115 of the 120 cases.

STRATIFIED ANALYSIS

Although it has been said that every epidemiologic study can be summarized in a two-by-two table, many such studies require more sophisticated analyses than those described so far in this chapter. For example, two different exposures may appear to be associated with disease. How do you analyze both at the same time? Even when you are only interested in the association of one particular exposure and one particular outcome, a third factor may complicate the association. The two princi-

Table 8–8. Food-Specific Attack Rates for Persons Who Ate Sunday Lunch, *Salmonella* Outbreak, South Carolina, 1990[a]

	ATE			DID NOT EAT					
FOOD	# CASES	TOTAL	AR %	# CASES	TOTAL	AR %	RR	(95% CI)	P VALUE
Turkey	115	204	56	5	41	12	4.6	(2.0, 10.6)	<0.001
Ham	65	121	54	54	122	44	1.2	(0.9, 1.6)	0.178
Dressing	99	186	53	21	59	36	1.5	(1.0, 2.2)	0.027
Gravy	85	159	53	35	85	41	1.3	(1.0, 1.7)	0.090
Macaroni	76	139	55	44	106	42	1.3	(1.0, 1.7)	0.056
Beans	96	183	52	23	61	38	1.4	(1.0, 2.0)	0.065
Corn	80	153	52	40	92	43	1.2	(0.9, 1.6)	0.229
Rolls	78	158	49	41	84	49	1.0	(0.8, 1.3)	0.958
Butter	47	88	53	73	157	46	1.2	(0.9, 1.5)	0.365
Tea	102	203	50	18	42	43	1.2	(0.8, 1.7)	0.482
Coffee	9	28	32	111	217	51	0.6	(0.4, 1.1)	0.090
Cranberries	42	74	57	78	171	46	1.2	(1.0, 1.6)	0.144

[a]AR indicates attack rate; RR, relative risk, and CI, confidence interval.
Source: Luby et al. (1993).[2]

pal types of complications are *confounding* and *effect modification*. Stratified analysis, which involves examining the exposure-disease association within different categories of a third factor, is one method for dealing with these complications.

Stratified analysis is an effective method for looking at the effects of two different exposures on the disease. Consider a hypothetical outbreak of hepatitis A among junior high school students. The investigators, not knowing the vehicle, administered a food consumption questionnaire to 50 students with hepatitis A and to 50 well controls. Two exposures had elevated odds ratios and statistically significant *P* values: milk and donuts (Table 8–9). Donuts were often consumed with milk, so many people were exposed to both or neither. How do you tease apart the effect of each item?

Stratification is one way to tease apart the effects of the two foods. First, decide which food will be the exposure of interest and which will be the stratification variable. Since donuts has the larger odds ratio, you might choose donuts as the primary exposure and milk as the stratification variable. The results are shown in Table 8–10. The odds ratio for donuts is 6.0, whether milk was consumed or not. Now, what if you had decided to look at the milk-illness association, stratified by donuts? Those results are shown in Table 8–11. Clearly, from Table 8–10, consumption of donuts remains strongly associated with disease, regardless of milk consumption. On the other hand, from Table 8–11, milk consumption is not independently associated with disease, with an odds ratio of 1.0 among those who did and did not eat donuts. Milk only *appeared* to be associated with illness because so many milk drinkers also ate donuts.

An alternative method for analyzing two exposures is with a two-by-four table, as shown in Table 8–12. In that table, exposure 1 is labeled "EXP 1"; exposure 2 is labeled "EXP 2." To calculate the risk ratio for each row, divide the attack rate ("risk") for that row by the attack rate for the group not exposed to either

Table 8–9. Hepatitis A and Consumption of Milk and Donuts

MILK	CASES	CONTROLS	TOTAL	
EXPOSED	37	21	58	Odds ratio = 3.9
UNEXPOSED	13	29	42	Yates-corrected χ^2 = 9.24
TOTAL	50	50	100	*P* value = 0.0002

DONUTS	CASES	CONTROLS	TOTAL	
EXPOSED	40	20	60	Odds ratio = 6.0
UNEXPOSED	10	30	40	Yates-corrected χ^2 = 15.04
	50	50	100	*P* value = 0.0001

Table 8–10. Hepatitis A and Donut Consumption, Stratified by Milk

		DRANK MILK					DID NOT DRINK MILK	
		CASES	CONTROLS				CASES	CONTROLS
ATE	YES	36	18		ATE	YES	4	2
DONUT?	NO	1	3		DONUT?	NO	9	27
		Odds ratio = 6.0					Odds ratio = 6.0	

Table 8–11. Hepatitis A and Milk Consumption, Stratified by Donuts

		ATE DONUT					DID NOT EAT DONUT	
		CASES	CONTROLS				CASES	CONTROLS
DRANK	YES	36	18		DRANK	YES	1	3
MILK?	NO	4	2		MILK?	NO	9	27
		Odds ratio = 1.0					Odds ratio = 1.0	

exposure (bottom row in Table 8–12). To calculate the odds ratio for each row, use that row's values for a and b in the usual formula, ad/bc.

With this presentation, it is easy to see the effect of exposure 1 alone (row 3) compared with the unexposed group (row 4), exposure 2 alone (row 2) compared with the unexposed group (row 4), and exposure 1 and 2 together (row 1) compared with the unexposed group (row 4). Thus the separate and joint effects can be assessed.

From Table 8–13, you can see that donuts alone had an odds ratio of 6.0, whereas milk alone had an odds ratio of 1.0. Together, donuts and milk had an odds ratio of 6.0, the same as donuts alone. In other words, donuts, but not milk,

Table 8–12. Data Layout for Two-by-Four Table, Analyzing Two Exposures at Once

EXP 1	EXP 2	ILL	WELL	TOTAL	RISK	RISK RATIO	ODDS RATIO
Yes	Yes	a_{YY}	b_{YY}	h_{YY}	a_{YY}/h_{YY}	$Risk_{YY}/Risk_{NN}$	$a_{YY}d/b_{YY}c$
No	Yes	a_{NY}	b_{NY}	h_{NY}	a_{NY}/h_{NY}	$Risk_{NY}/Risk_{NN}$	$a_{NY}d/b_{NY}c$
Yes	No	a_{YN}	b_{YN}	h_{YN}	a_{YN}/h_{YN}	$Risk_{YN}/Risk_{NN}$	$a_{YN}d/b_{YN}c$
No	No	c	d	h_{NN}	c/h_{NN}	1.0 (Ref)	1.0 (Ref)

Table 8–13. Hepatitis A and Consumption of Milk and Donuts,
in Two-by-Four Table Layout

DONUT	MILK	CASE	CONTROL	ODDS RATIO
Yes	Yes	36	18	6.0
No	Yes	1	3	1.0
Yes	No	4	2	6.0
No	No	9	27	1.0 (Ref)

were associated with illness. The two-by-four table summarizes the stratified tables
in one and eliminates the need to designate one of the foods as the primary exposure and the other as the stratification variable.

Confounding

Stratification also helps in the identification and handling of confounding. *Confounding is the distortion of an exposure-disease association by the effect of some
third factor (a "confounder").* A third factor may be a confounder and distort the
exposure-disease association if it is

- Associated with the outcome independent of the exposure—that is, even
  in the nonexposed group (In other words, it must be an independent "risk
  factor.")
- Associated with the exposure but not a consequence of it

To separate out the effect of the exposure from the effect of the confounder, stratify
by the confounder.

Consider the mortality rates in Alaska versus Arizona. In 1988, the crude
mortality rate in Arizona was 7.9 deaths per 1,000 population, over twice as high
as the crude mortality rate in Alaska (3.9 deaths per 1,000 population). Is living
in Arizona more hazardous to one's health? The answer is no. In fact, for most
age groups, the mortality rate in Arizona is about equal to or slightly lower than
the mortality rate in Alaska. The population of Arizona is older than the population of Alaska, and death rates rise with age. Age is a confounder that wholly
accounts for Arizona's apparently elevated death rate—the age-adjusted mortality rates for Arizona and Alaska are 7.5/1000 and 8.4/1000, respectively. Note
that age satisfies the two criteria described above: increasing age is associated with
increased mortality, regardless of where one lives; and age is associated with state
of residence (Arizona's population is older than Alaska's).

Return to the sequence in which an analysis should be conducted (Figure 8–1). After you have assessed the basic exposure-disease relationships using two-by-two tables, you should stratify the data by "third variables"—variables that are cofactors, potential confounders, or effect modifiers (described below). If your simple two-by-two table analysis has identified two or more possible risk factors, each should be stratified by the other or others. In addition, you should develop a list of other variables to be assessed. The list should include the known risk factors for the disease (one of the two criteria for a confounder) and matching variables. Then stratify or separate the data by categories of relevant third variables. For each stratum, compute a stratum-specific measure of association. Age is so often a real confounder that it is reasonable to consider it a potential confounder in almost any data set. Using age as an example, you could separate the data by 10-year age groups (strata), create a separate two-by-two table of exposure and outcome for each stratum, and calculate a measure of association for each stratum.

The result of this type of analysis is that, within each stratum, "like is compared with like." If the stratification variable is gender, then in one stratum the exposure-disease relationship can be assessed for women and in the other the same relationship can be assessed for men. Gender can no longer be a confounder in these strata, since women are compared with women and men are compared with men.

To look for confounding, first look at the smallest and largest values of the stratum-specific measures of association and compare them with the crude value. If the crude value does not fall within the range between the smallest and largest stratum-specific values, confounding is surely present.

Often, confounding is not quite that obvious. So the next step is to calculate a summary "adjusted" measure of association as a weighted average of the stratum-specific values. The most common method of controlling for confounding is by stratifying the data and then computing measures that represent weighted averages of the stratum-specific data. One popular technique was developed by Mantel and Haenszel. This and other methods are described in Reference 5. After calculating a summary value, compare the summary value to the crude value to see if the two are "appreciably different." Unfortunately, there are no hard-and-fast rules or statistical tests to determine what constitutes "appreciably different." In practice, we assume that the summary adjusted value is more accurate. The question then becomes, "Does the crude value adequately approximate the adjusted value, or would the crude value be misleading to a reader?" If the crude and adjusted values are close, you can use the crude because it is not misleading and it is easier to explain. If the two values are appreciably different (10 percent? 20 percent?), use the adjusted value.

After deciding whether the crude or adjusted or stratum-specific measures of association are appropriate, you can then perform hypothesis testing and calculate confidence intervals for the chosen measures.

Effect Modification

The third use of stratification is in assessing effect modification. *Effect modification* means, simply, that the degree of association between an exposure and an outcome differs in different subgroups of the population. For example, a measles vaccine (exposure) may be highly effective (strong association) in preventing disease (outcome) if given after a child is 15 months of age (stratification variable = age at vaccination, stratum 1 = ≥15 months), but less effective (weaker association) if given before 15 months (age stratum 2 = <15 months). As a second example, tetracycline (exposure) may cause (strong association) tooth mottling (outcome) among children (stratifier = age, stratum 1 = children), but tetracycline does not cause tooth mottling among adults. In both examples, the association or effect is a function of, or is modified by, some third variable. Effect modification is enlightening because it raises questions for further research. Why does the effect vary? In what way is one group different from the other? Studying these and related questions can lead to insights into pathophysiology, natural history of disease, and genetic or acquired host characteristics that influence risk.

Basically, evaluation for effect modification involves determining whether the stratum-specific measures of association differ from one another. Identification of effect modification is really a two-part process involving these questions:

1. Is the range of associations wide enough to be of public health or scientific importance? (A credo of field epidemiology is that "a difference, to be a difference, has to make a difference.")
2. Is the range of associations likely to represent normal sampling variation? Evaluation can be done either qualitatively ("eyeballing the results") or quantitatively (done with multivariate analysis such as logistic regression or with statistical tests of heterogeneity).

Another difference is important to note: confounding is extremely common because it is just an artifact of the data. True effect modification, on the other hand, usually represents a biological phenomenon and hence is much less common.

ADDITIONAL ANALYSES

Two additional areas are worth mentioning, although technical discussions are beyond the scope of this book. These two areas are the assessment of dose-response relationships and modeling.

Dose Response

In epidemiology, *dose-response* means increased risk of disease with increasing (or, for a protective exposure, decreasing) amount of exposure. Amount of exposure may reflect intensity of exposure (e.g., milligrams of L-tryptophan or number of cigarettes per day) or duration of exposure (e.g., number of months or years of exposure) or both.

If an association between an exposure and a health problem has been established, epidemiologists often take the next step to look for a dose-response effect. Indeed, the presence of a dose-response effect is one of the well-recognized criteria for inferring causation. Statistical techniques are available for assessing such relationships, even when confounders must be taken into account.

The first step, as always, is organizing your data. One convenient format is a 2-by-H table, where H represents the categories or doses of exposure.

As shown in Table 8–14, an odds ratio (or a risk ratio for a cohort study) can be calculated for each dose relative to the lowest dose or the unexposed group. You can calculate confidence intervals for each dose as well.

Merely eyeballing the data in this format can give you a sense of whether a dose-response relationship is present. If the odds ratios increase or decrease monotonically, a statistically significant dose-response relationship may be present. The Mantel extension test is one method of assessing the statistical significance of a dose-response effect. The mechanics of this test are described in Reference 6. The test yields a chi-square statistic with one degree of freedom.

Modeling

There comes a time in the life of many epidemiologists when neither simple nor stratified analysis can do justice to the data. At such times, epidemiologists may

Table 8–14. Data Layout and Notation for Dose-Response Table

	ILL	WELL		*Odds ratio*
Dose 5	a_5	b_5	h_5	$a_5 d/b_5 c$
Dose 4	a_4	b_4	h_4	$a_4 d/b_4 c$
Dose 3	a_3	b_3	h_3	$a_3 d/b_3 c$
Dose 2	a_2	b_2	h_2	$a_2 d/b_2 c$
Dose 1	a_1	b_1	h_1	$a_1 d/b_1 c$
Dose 0	c	d	h_0	1.0 (reference)
	v_1	v_0	t	

turn to modeling. Modeling is a technique of fitting the data to particular statistical equations. One group of models are regression models, where the outcome is a function of exposure variables, confounders, and interaction terms (effect modifiers). The types of data usually dictate the type of regression model that is most appropriate. For example, logistic regression is the model most epidemiologists choose for binary outcome variables (ill/well, case/control, alive/dead, etc.).

In logistic regression, a binary outcome (dependent) variable is modeled as a function of a series of independent variables. The independent variables should include the exposure or exposures of primary interest and may include confounders and more complex interaction terms. Software packages provide beta coefficients for each independent term. If the model includes only the outcome variable and the primary exposure variable coded as (0,1), then e^β should equal the odds ratio you could calculate from the two-by-two table. If other terms are included in the model, then e^β equals the odds ratio adjusted for all the other terms. Logistic regression can also be used to assess dose-response relationships, effect modification, and more complex relationships. A variant of logistic regression called conditional logistic regression is particularly appropriate for pair-matched data.

Other types of models used in epidemiology include Cox proportional hazards models for life-table analysis, binomial regression for risk ratio analysis, and Poisson regression for analysis of rare-event data.

Keep in mind that *sophisticated analytic techniques cannot atone for sloppy data*. Analytic techniques such as those described in this chapter are only as good as the data to which they are applied. Analytic techniques, whether they be simple, stratified, or multivariate, use the information at hand. They do not ask or assess whether the proper comparison group was selected, whether the response rate was adequate, whether exposure and disease were properly defined, or whether the data coding and entry were free of errors. Analytic techniques are merely tools; as the analyst, you are responsible for knowing the quality of the data and interpreting the results appropriately.

MATCHING IN CASE-CONTROL STUDIES

Early in this chapter we noted that different study designs require different analytic methods. Matching is one design that requires methods different from those described so far. Because matching is so common in field studies, this section addresses this important topic.

Matching generally refers to a case-control study design in which controls are intentionally selected to be similar to case-subjects on one or more specified characteristics (other than the exposure or exposures of interest). The goal of matching, like that of stratified analysis, is to "compare like with like." The characteristics most appropriately specified for matching are those that are potential confounders of the exposure-disease associations of interest. By matching cases and controls on factors such as age, gender, or geographic area, the distribution of those factors among cases and controls will be identical. In other words, the matching variable will not be associated with case-control status in the study. As a result, if the analysis is properly done, the matching variable will not confound the association of primary interest.

Two types of matching schemes are commonly used in epidemiology. One type is *pair matching*, where each control is selected according to its similarity to a *particular* case. This method is most appropriate when each case is unique in terms of the matching factor, for example, 50 cases widely scattered geographically. Each case could be matched to a friend or neighborhood control. That control is suitably matched to that particular case-subject, but not to any other case-subject in the study. The matching by design into these unique pairs must be maintained in the analysis.

The term "pair matching" is sometimes generalized to include not only matched pairs (case and one control), but matched triplets (case and two controls), quadruplets, and so on. The term also refers to studies in which the number of matched controls per case varies, so long as the controls are matched to a specific case.

The other type of matching is *category matching*, also called *frequency matching*. Category matching is a form of stratified sampling of controls, wherein controls are selected in proportion to the number of cases in each category of a matching variable. For example, in a study of 70 male and 30 female case-subjects, if 100 controls were also desired, you would select 70 male controls at random from the pool of all non-ill males and 30 female controls from the female pool. The pairs are not unique; any male control is a suitable match to any male case-subject. Data collected by category matching in the study design must be analyzed using stratified analysis.

Matching has several advantages. Matching on factors such as neighborhood, friendship, or sibship may control for confounding by numerous social factors that would be otherwise impossible to measure and control. Matching may be cost- and time-efficient, facilitating enrollment of controls. For example, matched friend controls may be identified while interviewing each case-subject, and these friends are more likely to cooperate than controls randomly selected from the general population. And finally, matching on a confounder increases the statistical efficiency of an analysis and thus provides narrower confidence intervals.

Matching has disadvantages, too. The primary disadvantage is that matching on a factor prevents you from examining its association with disease. If the age and gender distribution of case-subjects and controls are identical because you matched on those two factors, you cannot use your data to evaluate age and gender as risk factors themselves. Matching may be both cost- and time-inefficient, if considerable work must be performed to identify appropriately matched controls. The more variables to be matched on, the more difficult it will be to find suitably matched controls. In addition, matching on a factor that is not a confounder or having to discard cases because suitable controls could not be found decreases statistical efficiency and results in wider confidence intervals. Finally, matching complicates the analysis, particularly if other confounders are present.

In summary, matching is desirable and beneficial when you know beforehand that (1) you do not wish to examine the relationship between the matching factor and disease, (2) the factor is related to risk of disease so it is a potential confounder, and (3) matching is convenient or at least worth the potential extra costs to you. When in doubt, do not match, or match only on a strong risk factor that is likely to be distributed differently between exposed and unexposed groups and that is not a risk factor you are interested in assessing.

Matched Pairs

The basic data layout for a matched pair analysis appears at first glance to resemble the simple unmatched two-by-two tables presented earlier in this chapter, but in reality the two are quite different. In the matched-pair two-by-two table, each cell represents the number of matched pairs who meet the row and column criteria. In the unmatched two-by-two table, each cell represents the number of individuals who meet the criteria.

In Table 8–15, E+ denotes "exposed" and E– denotes "unexposed." Cell f thus represents the number of pairs made up of an exposed case and an unexposed control. Cells e and h are called *concordant pairs* because the case and control are in the same exposure category. Cells f and g are called *discordant pairs*.

In a matched-pair analysis, only the discordant pairs are informative. The odds ratio is computed as

$$\text{Odds ratio} = f \, / \, g$$

The test of significance for a matched pair analysis is the McNemar chi-square test. Both uncorrected and corrected formulas are commonly used.

$$\text{Uncorrected McNemar test} = \frac{(f - g)^2}{(f + g)}$$

$$\text{Corrected McNemar test} = \frac{(|f - g| - 1)^2}{(f + g)}$$

Table 8–15. Data Layout and Notation for Matched-Pair
Two-by-Two Table

		CONTROLS		
		E+	E–	Total
CASES	E+	e	f	e + f
	E–	g	h	g + h
	TOTAL	e + g	f + h	e + f + g + h

Table 8–16. Continual Tampon Use during
Index Menstrual Period in Case-Control Pairs,
Toxic Shock Syndrome Study, 1980

		CONTROLS		
		YES	NO	TOTAL
CASES	YES	33	9	42
	NO	1	1	2
	TOTAL	34	10	44 pairs

Odds ratio = 9 / 1 = 9.0

McNemar uncorrected chi-square test = $(9 - 1)^2 / (9 + 1) = 6.40$ $(P = 0.01)$

McNemar corrected chi-square test = $(|9 - 1| - 1)^2 / (9 + 1) = 4.90$ $(P = 0.03)$

Source: Shands et al. (1980).[7]

Table 8–16 presents the data from a pair-matched case-control study conducted in 1980 to assess the association between tampon use and toxic shock syndrome.[6]

Matched Triplets

The data layout for a study in which two controls are matched to each case is shown in Table 8–17. Each cell is named f_{ij}, where i is the number of exposed cases (1 if the case is exposed, 0 if the case is unexposed), and j is the number of exposed controls in the triplet. Thus cell f_{02} contains the number of triplets in which the case is unexposed but both controls are exposed.

A formula for calculating an odds ratio with *any* number of controls per case is

$$OR = \frac{\text{Number of unexposed controls matched with exposed cases}}{\text{Number of exposed controls matched with unexposed cases}}$$

For matched triplets, this formula reduces to

$$\text{Odds ratio} = \frac{2f_{10} + f_{11}}{2f_{02} + f_{01}}$$

Table 8–17 shows data from a case-control study of Kawasaki syndrome in Washington State.[8] For each of 16 cases-subjects, two age- and neighborhood-matched controls were identified. Although the study found no association with carpet cleaning, it did find the usual association with high household income (Table 8–18).

Larger Matched Sets and Variable Matching

Analogous analytic methods are available for matched sets of any fixed size and for sets with variable numbers of controls per case.[9] Such data are best analyzed with appropriate computer software, such as *Epi Info*.

Table 8–17. Data Layout and Notation for a Matched Case-Control Study with Two Controls per Case

		PERCENT EXPOSED CONTROLS		
		2 of 2	1 of 2	0 of 2
CASES	E+	f_{12}	f_{11}	f_{10}
	E−	f_{02}	f_{01}	f_{00}

Table 8–18. Kawasaki Syndrome and Annual Household Income > $40,000, Washington State, 1986

		NUMBER OF EXPOSED CONTROLS		
		2 of 2	1 of 2	0 of 2
CASES	E+	0	1	7
	E−	0	4	4

Odds ratio = $(2 \times 7 + 1) / (2 \times 0 + 4) = 3.8$

Source: Dicker (1986).[8]

Does a matched design require a matched analysis?

Does a matched design require a matched analysis? Usually, yes. In a pair-matched study, if the pairs are unique (siblings, friends, etc.), then pair-matched analysis is needed. If the pairs were based on a nonunique characteristic such as gender or race, stratified analysis is preferred. In a frequency matched study, stratified analysis is necessary.

In practice, some epidemiologists perform the appropriate matched analysis, then "break the match" and perform an unmatched analysis on the same data. If the results are similar, they may opt to present the data in unmatched fashion. In most instances, the unmatched odds ratio will be closer to 1.0 than the matched odds ratio ("bias toward the null"). Less frequently, the "broken" or unmatched odds ratio will be further from the null. These differences, which are related to confounding, may be trivial or substantial. The chi-square test result from unmatched data may be particularly misleading, usually being larger than the McNemar test result from the matched data. The decision to use a matched analysis or unmatched analysis is analogous to the decision to present crude or adjusted results. You must use your epidemiologic judgment in deciding whether the unmatched results are misleading to your audience or, worse, to yourself!

INTERPRETING FIELD DATA

> "Skepticism is the chastity of the intellect. . . .
> Don't give it away to the first attractive hypothesis that comes along."
>
> M. B. Gregg,
> after George Santayana

Does an elevated relative risk or odds ratio or a statistically significant chi-square test mean that the exposure is a true cause of disease? Certainly not. Although the association may indeed be causal, flaws in study design, execution, and analysis can result in apparent associations that are actually artifacts. Chance, selection bias, information bias, confounding, and investigator error should all be evaluated as possible explanations for an observed association.

One possible explanation for an observed association is chance. Under the null hypothesis, you assume that your study population is a sample from some source population and that incidence of disease is not associated with exposure in the source population. The role of chance is assessed through the use of tests of statistical significance. (As noted above, confidence intervals can be used as well.) A very small P value indicates that the null hypothesis is an *unlikely* explanation of the result you found. Keep in mind that chance can never be ruled out entirely—even if the P value is small, say 0.01. Yours may be the one sample in a hundred in which the null hypothesis is true and chance *is* the explanation! Note that tests of significance only evaluate the role of chance. They do not say anything about the roles of selection bias, information bias, confounding, or investigator error, discussed below.

Another explanation for the observed explanation is selection bias. *Selection bias* is a systematic error in the study groups or in the enrollment of study participants that results in a mistaken estimate of an exposure's effect on the risk of disease. In more simplistic terms, selection bias may be thought of as a problem arising from who gets into the study. Selection bias may arise either in the design or in the execution of the study. Selection bias may arise from the faulty design of a case-control study if, for example, too loose a case definition is used (so some persons in the case group do not actually have the disease being studied), asymptomatic cases go undetected among the controls, or an inappropriate control group is used. In the execution phase, selection bias may result if eligible subjects with certain exposure and disease characteristics choose not to participate or cannot be located. For example, if ill persons with the exposure of interest know the hypothesis of the study and are more willing to participate than other ill persons, then cell a in the two-by-two table will be artificially inflated compared to cell c, and the odds ratio will also be inflated. So to evaluate the possible role of selection bias, you must look at how cases and controls were specified and how they were enrolled.

Another possible explanation of an observed association is information bias. *Information bias* is a systematic error in the collection of exposure or outcome data about the study participants that results in a mistaken estimate of an exposure's effect on the risk of disease. Again, in more simplistic terms, information bias is a problem with the information you collect from the people in the study. Information bias may arise in a number of ways, including poor wording or understanding of a question on a questionnaire, poor recall (what did YOU have for lunch a week ago Tuesday?), or inconsistent interviewing technique. Information bias may also arise if a subject knowingly provides false information, either to hide the truth or, as is common in some cultures, in an attempt to please the interviewer.

As discussed earlier in this chapter, confounding can also distort an association. To evaluate the role of confounding, ensure that a list of potential confounders has been drawn up, that they have been evaluated for confounding, and that they have been controlled for as necessary.

Finally, investigator error has been known to be the explanation for some apparent associations. A missed button on a calculator, an erroneous transcription of a value, or use of the wrong formula can all yield artifactual associations! Check your work, or have someone else try to replicate it.

So before considering whether an association may be causal, consider whether the association may be explained by chance, selection bias, information bias, confounding, or investigator error. Now suppose that an elevated risk ratio or odds ratio has a small P value and narrow confidence interval, so chance is an unlikely explanation. Specification of cases and controls is reasonable and participation was good, so selection bias is an unlikely explanation. Information was collected using a standard questionnaire by an experienced and well-trained interviewer. Confounding by other risk factors was assessed and found not to be present or to have been controlled for. Data entry and calculations were verified. But before you conclude that the association is causal, you should consider the strength of the association, its biological plausibility, consistency with results from other studies, temporal sequence, and dose-response relationship, if any.

Strength of the association

In general, the stronger the association, the more likely one is to believe it is real. Thus we are generally more willing to believe that a relative risk of 9.0 may be causal than a relative risk of 1.5. This is not to say that a relative risk of 1.5 cannot reflect a causal relationship; it can. It is just that a subtle selection bias, information bias, or confounding could easily account for a relative risk of 1.5. The bias would have to be quite dramatic to account for a relative risk of 9.0!

Biological plausibility

Does the association make sense? Is it consistent with what is known of the pathophysiology, the known vehicles, the natural history of disease, animal models, or other relevant biological factors? For an implicated food vehicle in an infectious disease outbreak, can the agent be identified in the food, or will the agent survive (or even thrive) in the food? While some outbreaks are caused by new or previously unrecognized vehicles or risk factors, most are caused by those that we already know.

Consistency with other studies

Are the results consistent with those from other studies? A finding is more plausible if it can be replicated by different investigators, using different methods in different populations.

Exposure precedes disease

This criterion seems obvious, but in a retrospective study it may be difficult to document that exposure precedes disease. Suppose, for example, that persons with a particular type of leukemia are more likely to have antibodies to a particular virus. It might be tempting to conclude that the virus causes the leukemia, but from the serologic evidence at hand you could not be certain that exposure to the virus preceded the onset of leukemic changes.

Dose-response effect

Evidence of a dose-response effect adds weight to the evidence for causation. A dose-response effect is not a *necessary* feature for a relationship to be causal; some causal relationships may exhibit a threshold effect, for example. In addition, a dose-response effect does not rule out the possibility of confounding. Nevertheless, it is usually thought to add credibility to the association.

In many field investigations, a likely culprit may not meet all the criteria listed above. Perhaps the response rate was less than ideal, or the etiologic agent could not be isolated from the implicated food, or the dose-response analysis was inconclusive. Nevertheless, if the public's health is at risk, failure to meet every criterion should not be used as an excuse for inaction. As stated by George Comstock, "The art of epidemiologic reasoning is to draw sensible conclusions from imperfect data."[10] After all, field epidemiology is a tool for public health action to promote and protect the public's health based on science (sound epidemiologic methods), causal reasoning, and a healthy dose of practical common sense.

> "All scientific work is incomplete—whether it be observational or experimental. All scientific work is liable to be upset or modified by advancing knowledge. That does not confer upon us a freedom to ignore the knowledge we already have, or to postpone the action it appears to demand at a given time."[11]
>
> Sir Austin Bradford Hill

APPENDIX 8-1. FISHER EXACT TEST

The probability that the value in cell "a" is equal to the observed value, under the null hypothesis, is

$$Pr(a) = \frac{(v_1)!\,(v_0)!\,(h_1)!\,(h_0)!}{t!\,a!\,b!\,c!\,d!}$$

where k! ("k factorial") = $1 \times 2 \times \ldots \times k$,
(e.g., $5! = 1 \times 2 \times 3 \times 4 \times 5 = 120$)

The easiest way to compute a two-tailed Fisher exact test is compute a one-tailed test and multiply by 2. Computing the one-tailed test is the hard part!

To compute the one-tailed Fisher exact test, first calculate the exact probability that cell a equals the observed value, using the formula shown above. Next, keeping all of the row and column totals the same, add or subtract 1 to the observed value in cell a to get a value even more extreme than the value observed. Modify the values in the other cells as necessary (add or subtract 1 to get the right row and column totals), and use the formula shown above to compute this new value's exact probability. Continue adding or subtracting 1 and computing probabilities until no more extreme values are possible without changing the marginal totals. Finally, sum these individual probabilities to get the one-tailed P value. For a two-tailed P value, add any smaller probabilities from the other tail.

Example

	ILL	WELL	TOTAL	
EXPOSED	4	17	21	Odds ratio = undefined
UNEXPOSED	0	19	19	(cannot divide by zero)
TOTAL	4	36	40	

Based on the margins of this two-by-two table, cell a can take on values from 0 to 4, but none more extreme than 4. The probabilities for each value from 0 to 4 are

a	b	c	d	Probability	
4	17	0	19	4!36!21!19! / 40!4!17!0!19!	= 0.07
3	18	1	18	4!36!21!19! / 40!3!18!1!18!	= 0.28
2	19	2	17	4!36!21!19! / 40!2!19!2!17!	= 0.39
1	20	3	16	4!36!21!19! / 40!1!20!3!16!	= 0.22
0	21	4	15	4!36!21!19! / 40!0!21!4!15!	= 0.04.

Since there are no possible values of cell a more extreme than 4, the one-tailed P value is simply 0.07. The two-tailed P value is 0.07 + 0.04 = 0.11. Given a cutoff of 0.05, we could not reject the null hypothesis.

APPENDIX 8-2.

Chi-Square Table

DEGREE OF FREEDOM	PROBABILITY						
	0.50	0.20	0.10	0.05	0.02	0.01	0.001
1	0.455	1.642	2.706	3.841	5.412	6.635	10.827
2	1.386	3.219	4.605	5.991	7.824	9.210	13.815
3	2.366	4.642	6.251	7.815	9.837	11.345	16.268
4	3.357	5.989	7.779	9.488	11.668	13.277	18.465
5	4.351	7.289	9.236	11.070	13.388	15.086	20.517
10	9.342	13.442	15.987	18.307	21.161	23.209	29.588
15	14.339	19.311	22.307	24.996	28.259	30.578	37.697
20	19.337	25.038	28.412	31.410	35.020	37.566	43.315
25	24.337	30.675	34.382	37.652	41.566	44.314	52.620
30	29.336	36.250	40.256	43.773	47.962	50.892	59.703

Note: The Pearson chi-square test and the Yates corrected chi-square test from a two-by-two table have one degree of freedom. The Mantel-Haenszel chi-square also has one degree of freedom, whether from a single two-by-two table or from stratified analysis.

REFERENCES

1. Shem, S. (1978). *The house of God*. Richard Marek Publishers, New York.
2. Luby, S. P., Jones, J. L., Horan, J. M. (1993). A large salmonellosis outbreak catered by a frequently penalized restaurant. *Epidemiology and Infection*, 110, 31–39.
3. Berkelman, R. L., Martin, D., Graham, D. R., et al. (1982). Streptococcal wound infections caused by a vaginal carrier. *Journal of the American Medical Association*, 247, 2680–82.
4. Landrigan, P. J. (1972). Epidemic measles in a divided city. *Journal of the American Medical Association*, 221, 567–70.
5. Kleinbaum, D. G., Kupper, L. L., Morgenstern, H. (1982). *Epidemiologic research: principles and quantitative methods*. Lifetime Learning Publications, Belmont, California.
6. Schlesselman, J. J. (1982). *Case control studies: Design, conduct, analysis*. Oxford University Press, New York.
7. Shands, K. N., Schmid, G. P., Dan, B. B., et al. (1980). Toxic-shock syndrome in menstruating women: Association with tampon use and *Staphylococcus aureus* and clinical features in 52 cases. *New England Journal of Medicine*, 303, 1436–42.
8. Dicker, R. C. (1986). Kawasaki syndrome. *Washington Morbidity Report*,(Oct);1–4.
9. Robins, J., Greenland, S., Breslow, N. E. (1986). A general estimator for the variance of the Mantel-Haenszel odds ratio. *American Journal of Epidemiology*, 124, 719–23.
10. Comstock, G. W. (1990). Vaccine evaluation by case-control or prospective studies. *American Journal of Epidemiology*, 131, 205–207.
11. Hill, A. B. (1965). The environment and disease: Association or causation? *Proceedings of the Royal Society of Medicine*, 58, 295–300.

9

DEVELOPING INTERVENTIONS

Richard A. Goodman

James W. Buehler

Jeffrey P. Koplan

Epidemiologic field investigations are often done in response to acute public health problems. When outbreaks of disease occur, there is usually an urgent need to identify the source and/or cause of the problem as a basis for initiating control measures or other interventions. Alternatively, the identification of environmental or occupational hazards frequently demands an evaluation of exposed persons and an assessment of the risks of disease. Regardless of the nature of such problems, however, there will be an immediate need to investigate, to recommend control and preventive measures, and to convince the affected community to accept public health recommendations.

When circumstances require an immediate response, you must sometimes take and/or recommend specific public health actions without incontrovertible epidemiologic evidence of a causal relation. Under such circumstances, the key issue for the epidemiologist and the public health decision maker is represented by the following question: To what extent must an acute health problem be epidemiologically defined and understood before action is initiated? This chapter outlines factors that influence the conduct of epidemiologic field investigations and the decisions about interventions.

This chapter was adapted, with permission of the editors from Goodman, R. A., Buehler, J. W., Koplan, J. P. (1990). The epidemiologic field investigation: Science and judgment in public health practice. *American Journal of Epidemiology*, 132, 91–96.[1]

REASONS FOR INITIATING FIELD INVESTIGATIONS

In addition to the need to develop and implement control measures to end threats to the public's health, other reasons for field investigations include (1) program considerations such as available resources, (2) opportunities for research, (3) political and public concerns, (4) legal obligations, and (5) training.

Program Considerations

Certain disease-control programs at national, state, and local levels have specific and extensive requirements for epidemiologic investigation. For example, as part of the measles elimination effort in the United States, a measles outbreak is considered to exist in a community whenever one case of measles is confirmed.[2] Accordingly, every case of measles is investigated in order to identify and vaccinate susceptible persons and to evaluate such other control strategies as the exclusion from school of those children who cannot provide proof of immunity. A potentially detrimental effect of such policies is that costly investigations may yield limited public health benefit—as illustrated by the investigation of a single case of cholera in Texas in 1972.[3]

Because field investigations can be costly in personnel time and resources, they may detract from other activities. Thus, the capacity to do fieldwork may be limited by competing demands of other programs within an agency, whether at national, state, or local levels. Under these circumstances, failure to investigate a specific problem could result in a public health problem of greater magnitude, which, if controlled earlier, would have caused less economic loss.

Research Opportunities

Because outbreaks are "natural experiments," they also present opportunities to address questions of importance to investigators. Even when there is a clear policy for control of a specific problem, investigation may still provide opportunities to identify risk factors for infection or disease, define the clinical spectrum of disease, measure the impact of control measures or clinical interventions, or assess the usefulness of microbiological markers.

Some outbreaks that initially appear to be "routine" may lead to important epidemiologic discoveries. In 1983, for example, investigators pursued a cluster of diarrhea cases, an extremely common problem, to extraordinary lengths.[4] As a result, they were able to trace the chain of transmission of a unique strain of multiply antibiotic resistant *Salmonella* back from the affected persons to hamburger they consumed, to the meat supplier, and ultimately to the specific animal herd source. This investigation played a key role in clarifying the linkage between antibiotic use by the cattle industry and disease in humans.

Political and Public Concern

Although the public's perceptions of hazards may differ from those of epidemiologists, these perceptions sometimes drive the political process that mandates investigations or actions. In some cases, public concerns mandate investigations that are premature or unlikely to be fruitful from a scientific perspective but which are critical in terms of community relations. Small clusters of disease (e.g., leukemia or adverse fetal outcomes) are an example of problems that frequently generate great public concern. Small cluster outbreaks often occur by chance alone and only occasionally yield new research information when investigated.[5] However, because community members may perceive a health threat and because certain clusters do represent specific preventable risks, some public health agencies have developed standard procedures for investigating such clusters even though the likelihood of identifying a remediable cause is low.

At the other extreme, attempts at more thorough epidemiologic investigations can be misinterpreted as community experimentation or bureaucratic delay. In a large *Escherichia coli* enteric disease outbreak at Crater Lake National Park in 1975, a 1-day delay in implementing control measures to obtain more epidemiologic data resulted in a congressional hearing and charges of a "cover up."[6]

Legal Obligations

Some epidemiologic investigations are likely to be used as testimony in civil or criminal trials. In these situations, investigations may be carried further than they would be otherwise. For example, in an investigation of a cluster of cardiac arrests in an intensive care unit in Maryland in 1986, the investigation went to the unusual length of attempting to determine the contents of charts that could not be located.[7,8]

Training

By analogy to clerkships in medical school and postgraduate residencies, outbreak investigations provide opportunities for training in basic epidemiologic skills. Just as clinical training is often accomplished at the same time as patient care is provided, training in field epidemiology often simultaneously assists in disease control and prevention. For example, the Epidemic Intelligence Service program at CDC has provided assistance to state and local health departments while simultaneously training health professionals in the practice of applied epidemiology.[9]

DETERMINANTS FOR INTERVENTIONS

The severity of a specific problem is a key determinant of the urgency and course of a field investigation. Severity is indicated by correlates such as the degree and nature of complications (e.g., mortality), duration of illness, need for treatment and hospitalization, and economic impact. For example, virtually all cases of rabies occurring in humans in the United States trigger extensive epidemiologic investigations because of the vital need to prevent deaths by quickly identifying other exposures and the animal source. Similarly, nosocomial infection clusters—especially those in postsurgical or immunocompromised patients—are often investigated both because of the potential for serious complications and greatly prolonged hospitalization and the possibility of iatrogenic illness, with its own special urgency as an unnecessary medical event.

In addition to the severity of a problem, a spectrum of other factors influence the aggressiveness, extent, and scientific rigor of an epidemiologic field investigation. In the prototypical investigation, control measures are formulated only after a series of other steps have been carried out (see Chapter 5). In practice, however, decisions regarding control measures may be appropriate at any step in the sequence.

For most outbreaks of acute disease, the scope of an investigation is dictated by the levels of certainty about (1) the etiology of the problem (e.g., the specific pathogen or toxic agent) and (2) the source and/or mode of spread (e.g., water- or airborne). When the problem is identified, the levels of certainty regarding the etiology, source, mode of spread may range from known to unknown (Figure 9–1). These basic dichotomies are illustrated in the figure by four examples that probably represent the extremes.

In many situations, control measures can be implemented empirically; in others, interventions are appropriate only after exhaustive epidemiologic investigation. Often preliminary control measures can be started based on limited, initial information and then can be modified as investigations proceed. For example, the occurrence of a single case of hepatitis A in a day care center may lead to the administration of immune globulin prophylaxis to an entire cohort of exposed children and staff.[10] In this instance, the response is predicated on routine policy and guidelines that have been developed by experts based on studies, previous outbreak experience, and virtual certainty about both the etiology of the problem and its mode of spread.

More commonly, there is some degree of uncertainty about the etiology or about sources and the mode of spread (Figure 9–1). In most outbreaks of gastrointestinal disease, the control measures selected will depend on knowing whether transmission has resulted from person-to-person spread or from a common-source exposure and, if the latter, identifying the source. For example, an outbreak of

Source/transmission mode

		Known	Unknown
Etiology	**Known**	Investigation + Control +++ Example: Hepatitis A in a day care	Investigation +++ Control + Example: Salmonella in marijuana
	Unknown	Investigation +++ Control +++ Example: Parathion poisoning	Investigation +++ Control + Example: Legionnaires' disease

Figure 9–1. Relative emphasis of investigative and control efforts (response options) in disease outbreaks as influenced by levels of certainty about etiology and source/mode of transmission. "Investigation" means extent of the investigation; "control" means the basis for rapid implementation of control measures. Pluses show the level of response indicated: + = low; ++ = intermediate; +++ = high. *Source:* Goodman et al. (1990).[1]

Salmonella muenchen in several states in 1981 required an extensive epidemiologic field investigation, including an analytic (case-control) study, before the mode of spread was found to be personal use or household exposure to marijuana.[11] The converse situation (i.e., in which the source is presumed but the etiology is unknown) is illustrated by the nationwide outbreak of eosinophilia-myalgia syndrome in the United States in 1989.[12] In that outbreak, L-tryptophan, a dietary supplement, was initially implicated as the source of the exposure and provided material for subsequent laboratory analysis to define the actual agent. Finally, as illustrated by the legionnaires' disease outbreak in 1976, an extensive field investigation can fail to identify the cause, the source, and mode in time to control the acute problem but still enables advances in knowledge that ultimately lead to preventive measures.[13]

CAUSATION AND THE FIELD INVESTIGATION

The need to determine whether a statistical association also supports a causal relation is as essential to an epidemiologic field investigation as it is to a planned prospective study. Thus, the criteria to assess causal associations[14,15] are integral to the scientific framework of field investigations. The challenge to the public sector epidemiologist is to balance the need to assess causality through the process of scientific inquiry with the potentially conflicting need to intervene quickly to protect the public's health. Few epidemiologic field investigations appear to address the criteria of causality explicitly, because when the criteria are applied to such investigations, they may be only partially attained.

The usefulness of individual criteria (e.g., temporality, strength of association, biological gradient, consistency, plausibility) varies.[15] In any outbreak, multiple groups of persons may be exposed, affected, or involved in some respect. Because of differences in knowledge, beliefs, and perceived impact of the outbreak, each group may draw different conclusions regarding causality from the same information. For example, in a restaurant-associated food-borne outbreak, restaurant patrons, management, media, attorneys, and local health officials are each likely to have a different threshold for judging the food from the restaurant to be the source of disease. In this situation, the epidemiologist's concerns might focus on strength of association and biological gradient between exposure to a certain food item and illness, while a restaurant patron's primary concern may simply be plausibility. Attorneys, on the other hand, defending a restaurant epidemiologically associated with a food-borne epidemic, will often review the patients one by one. Their hope is to show that, with each case, there can be reasonable doubt that illness truly resulted from eating at the restaurant in question. By such tactics they hope to show that there was no epidemic.

SUMMARY

Epidemiologic field investigations are usually initiated in response to epidemics or the occurrence of other acute disease, injury, or environmental health problems. Under such circumstances, the primary objective of the field investigation will be to employ the scientific principles of epidemiology to determine a rational and appropriate response for ending or controlling the problem. Key factors that influence decisions regarding the timing and choice of public health interventions include the severity of the problem, levels of certainty about both the etiology and source of the problem, and the extent to which causal criteria have been established.

REFERENCES

1. Goodman, R. A., Buehler, J. W., and Koplan, J. P. (1990). The epidemiologic field investigation: Science and judgment in public health practice. *American Journal of Epidemiology*, 132, 91–96.
2. Centers for Disease Control (1987). Measles prevention. *Morbidity and Mortality Weekly Report*, 36, 409–26.
3. Weissman, J. B., DeWitt, W. E., Thompson, J., et al. (1975). A case of cholera in Texas, 1973. *American Journal of Epidemiology*, 100, 487–98.

4. Holmberg, S. D., Osterholm, M. T., Senger, K. A., et al. (1984). Drug-resistant *Salmonella* from animals fed antimicrobials. *New England Journal of Medicine*, 311, 617–22.

5. Schulte, P. A., Ehrenberg, R. L., Singal, M. (1987). Investigation of occupational cancer clusters: Theory and practice. *American Journal of Public Health*, 77, 52–56.

6. Rosenberg, M. L., Koplan, J. P., Wachsmith, I. K., et al. (1977). Epidemic diarrhea at Crater Lake from enterotoxigenic *Escherichia coli*: A large waterborne outbreak. *Annals of Internal Medicine*, 86, 714–18.

7. Sacks, J. J., Stroup, D. F., Will, M. L., et al. (1988). A nurse-associated epidemic of cardiac arrests in an intensive care unit. *Journal of the American Medical Association*, 259, 689–95.

8. Sacks, J. J., Aung, H. K., Sniezek, J. S. (1988). The epidemiology of missing records [letter]. *Journal of the American Medical Association*, 259, 685.

9. Thacker, S. B., Goodman, R. A., Dicker, R. C. (1990). Training and service in public health practice, 1951–90—CDC's Epidemic Intelligence Service. *Public Health Reports*, 105, 599–604.

10. Centers for Disease Control (1985). Recommendations for protection against viral hepatitis. *Morbidity and Mortality Weekly Report*, 34, 313–16.

11. Taylor, D. N., Wachsmuth, K., Yung-Hui, S., et al. (1982). Salmonellosis associated with marijuana: A multistate outbreak traced by plasmic fingerprinting. *New England Journal of Medicine*, 306, 1249–53.

12. Kilbourne, E. M. (1992). Eosinophilia-myalgia syndrome: Coming to grips with a new illness. *Epidemiologic Reviews*, 14, 16–36.

13. Fraser, D. W., Tsai, T. R., Orenstein, W., et al. (1977). Legionnaires' disease: Description of an epidemic of pneumonia. *New England Journal of Medicine* 297, 1189–97.

14. Hill, A. B. (1965). The environment and diseases: Association of causation? *Proceedings of the Royal Society of Medicine*, 58, 295–300.

15. Rothman, K. J. (1986). *Modern epidemiology*, pp. 16–20. Little, Brown and Company, Boston.

10

COMMUNICATING EPIDEMIOLOGIC FINDINGS

Michael B. Gregg

WRITING AN EPIDEMIOLOGIC PAPER

Among the skills of a good field epidemiologist is knowing how to communicate effectively. This chapter deals with some of the elements of both written and oral communication skills.

The single most important lesson to take home on this subject is that the data you collect are no more useful to fellow scientists and the public than your ability to communicate these findings convincingly.[1] Meaningful transfer of facts and their implications shapes medical and public health practice and determines the need to acquire new data. Therefore, communication stands as a prime function of the field epidemiologist.

A key word here is "convince." Chief Justice Oliver Wendell Holmes once said "A page of history is worth a volume of logic." What Justice Holmes meant was that if you want to move people to act, past experiences, real-life illustrations, and present-day success stories are much more persuasive than spelling out a series of logical analyses that tend to be cold, academic, and distant from everyday experience.

Another quotation from a famous American epidemiologist may also bring to light some of the more fundamental aspects of communicating epidemiologic findings. In defining epidemiology, Wade Hampton Frost, considered by many the "father" of American epidemiology, wrote, "Epidemiology is something more than the total of its established facts. It includes the orderly arrangement of fact into chains of inference that extend more or less beyond the bounds of direct observation." This tells us at least two things: first, that good epidemiology includes putting information into sensible order and, second, that the whole may be greater than the sum of the parts. Thus, once you assemble all the components, you may be able to draw more inferences from the aggregate than would appear to be possible when each fact is interpreted separately.

Basic Structure

Although varying somewhat from journal to journal, most formats of scientific papers include an introduction, a materials and methods section, and sections for results, discussion (or comment), and conclusions. Some articles have a summary and most have an abstract of the article at the very beginning. Sometimes, particularly in epidemiologic papers, there is a background section. The *Journal of the American Medical Association* (*JAMA*) has recently changed its abstract to include subheadings such as "Objective," "Design," "Setting," "Participants," "Interventions," "Main Outcome Measures," "Results," and "Conclusions." These divisions can be helpful in the overall organization of an epidemiologic paper.[2]

However, let us look at each one of these major sections briefly in order to get some ideas of their function.

Introduction

The introduction of virtually all scientific papers gives a very brief historical perspective. Epidemiologic papers are no exception. One should usually give some indication of why the investigation was done (i.e., because of an outbreak of illness or an apparent need to explain or explore why health events happened). One should also indicate the overall purpose of the paper and give some indication of the specific area to be covered. If the topic is cancer or outbreaks of *Salmonella* infection, say what particular facet will be emphasized. Look at published papers of that journal to get the acceptable format.

The introduction is not a literature review. You should pick out only the pertinent material and try to guide the reader's thinking into your own thought processes—where you are going and what will be encountered along the way.

Materials and methods

Tell the reader what tools and methods you used, how they were applied, and what you did, what the design of the study was, what operations were performed, and what rules and definitions were used in the investigation.

In an epidemiologic paper, a case definition is an absolute necessity because, if the readers do not know your definition, they do not know exactly what you are counting. Describe the case-finding techniques—contacting physicians, visiting all relevant clinics, doing a survey, analyzing an existing database, or various other methods of case finding. Outline the laboratory methods, but probably not in great detail in an epidemiologic paper. Describe surveys or other sampling techniques used, statistical tests applied, and any allied areas such as animal or vector studies and environmental characteristics.

Also, a statement concerning background or setting may fit appropriately here. Describe the area under investigation, the size of the community, or the scope of the hospital. Give the reader a denominator: "The community hospital served a population of 24,000 people," "There were 200 discharges per month," or "The community has a maximum population of 15,000 people, most of whom are migrant workers who come in during the peak harvesting season." Some detail about geographic, climatic, or physical features of where the investigation took place may be necessary. What was there when the investigation started and who was there? Key people may need to be identified (usually by title rather than by name). Such a section can also appear as part of the introduction or even be included in the results. After the first drafts of the paper are prepared, you will almost certainly have a better feeling of where a background statement best belongs.

Results

For a field investigation, the "results" section very often but not always starts with how the problem or epidemic was recognized and a very short description of the pertinent time, place, person findings. Such a short paragraph prepares the reader, giving a feeling of time moving and a sense of the whole picture—important components of good communication.

Now comes the first major area of the results: *descriptive epidemiology*. Start with the clinical and laboratory aspects first. Usually, there will be range of disease presentations, so describe the clinical findings in some detail. They will give the more clinically oriented reader an idea of the spectrum of disease and will often help justify the case definition. State what laboratory tests were done and their results. Avoid the tendency to defend the methods or to interpret the results at this point; that follows later in the discussion.

Next, in whatever detail is necessary, orient the reader to the time, place, and person of the investigation. This may involve considerable discussion about the timing and distribution of cases. It is the logical place to show an epidemic curve if appropriate. Describe the figure and analyze it for the reader. Then describe the findings according to place of occurrence and pertinent characteristics of the cases (age, gender, race, occupation, etc.). This section is still descriptive, but it should be as detailed as needed to help build the best possible foundation for the subsequent analysis. Include, if possible, pertinent negative findings. Such data are often as important as "positive" data and can materially help lead readers in the direction you want them to go. You are not doing any real analysis yet but are setting the scene to do so.

Next comes the *transition of thought* between descriptive and analytic epidemiology. This can often be a difficult task, particularly for the neophyte. Essentially, you are now taking the readers by the hand and leading them through an objective interpretation of the clinical, laboratory, and epidemiologic descriptive data. Guide them down plausible avenues of inference that can be considered and discarded or considered and established as the most reasonable and defensible explanation for what was found. Present the pertinent information in an orderly way, blending the findings and existing knowledge together in a persuasive path of logic. A possible order of considerations might be the following:

- What health problem (disease) do the clinical and laboratory data confirm or support?
- What do the facts of time, place, and person suggest?

And, almost simultaneously:

- How well does the existing knowledge of this disease's pathogenesis and epidemiology fit with the investigative findings? Can these facts help one understand or suggest what happened?
- What possible exposures occurred and how can one postulate a chain of events happening that would explain the health problem?
- What hypotheses come to mind?

Here is an example in a somewhat truncated form. *Descriptive facts*: In August 1980, a community hospital in Michigan recognized 7 cases of streptococcal wound infection in post-operative patients spanning the previous 4 months. Since this represented more cases than usual, an investigation was begun.[3] A total of 10 cases of streptococcal infection, all of the same serotype, were found over this time period. All were in patients on several surgical wards. *Transition*: The temporal and geographic clustering of cases, the fact that all infections developed within 1 to 2 days after surgery, and the fact that all infectious were of the same serotype strongly suggested a common exposure—presumably in the operating rooms. Since most streptococcal infectious in the hospital setting are transmitted by humans, the field team hypothesized that contact with or exposure to a member of the hospital staff posed the unique risk to the infected patients.

This example shows how the descriptive data plus a knowledge of the epidemiology of the infectious agent were combined to lead the reader, one would hope, to the same logical hypothesis as the investigators.

Now comes *analytic epidemiology*—that is, comparisons of cases and controls or those exposed and not exposed. If there were no apparent associations, one would probably not be writing the paper. If there were associations, what are the probabilities of them occurring? Here you will logically select risks and/or exposures that you compared and will present them to the reader. Consider starting with those comparisons that showed no statistically significant differences, then lead on to those where differences were noted and dwell on them.

To continue with the above example: the field team then compared infected patients to comparable noninfected postsurgical patients with respect to contact with 38 surgeons, anesthesiologists, and nursing staff. Rates of exposure to various hospital staff were not statistically different between cases and controls except for one nurse. The nurse was then found to be a carrier of the epidemic strain of *Streptococcus*. When she was removed from the surgical wards, no more cases of streptococcal infection occurred.

Sometimes the first analyses reveal nothing requiring another level of analysis and/or collection of new data. This is particularly characteristic of nosocomial infections, where numbers of cases are often small, as in the outbreak above. In any event take your reader, logically, step by step through your analyses.

If control and/or prevention measures were taken, this is the place to include them in the paper.

Discussion

A good discussion highlights the significant findings without reviewing everything all over again. The most salient points can be restated for emphasis. You can now express your own judgment as to what the results mean and show how your findings relate to the current state of knowledge. You should weigh the possible implications of all of your data as you go along, and then you should give your judgment in terms of a conclusion.

Be sure to review the definitions, measurements, and analytic tools that you used (e.g., case definitions, survey instruments, levels of sensitivity and specificity, and statistical tests). How good were they? Were they the most appropriate instruments for the study? Weigh them fairly for the readers so that they know how you view them. What were the weaknesses or difficulties you had in collecting important information? Did lack of relevant data have a significant impact with regard to confounding or effect modification?

Be a critic of your methods, yet defend them objectively and honestly. You will be much more believable if you do so. Exactly where in the discussion you include these remarks will depend a great deal upon their importance in verifying your findings. In fact, you may want to discuss the pros and cons of your methods as you interpret the findings. In general, however, evaluations of methods will fall after the major points of the discussion.

Conclusion

Summarize the results and inferences of the work in one short paragraph. You may also want to include in a sentence or two what further work or research is needed to clarify or expand the findings of your study.

Order of Writing

Let us next talk about the sequence you might consider in starting to write an article. You have done the investigation and you know the component parts; how do you now begin to draft the article? The temptation is clearly to start at the beginning, namely, the introduction, and continue to the end. Consider avoiding this temptation and describe the facts first. It is a much more comfortable process. Some fledgling authors spend a great deal of time and effort spinning their wheels trying to write an introduction, not knowing how much of the literature to review, not yet knowing what their major points are going to be, not knowing how they want to orient the reader. So forget about the introduction; sit down and write about what you did and what you found—that is, what you know as nobody else knows.

So consider writing the body of the study—the background, the materials and methods, and the results—first. The discussion and introduction will still be there waiting and may appear in a better perspective if you first write about what you did and what you found out. Also, you will have exercised your descriptive and analytic mind, so that by the time the discussion, the introduction, and the conclusion are ready to be written, you will see the major and minor findings quite clearly. In truth, you may not really be aware of some of the key issues, the new facts and their ramifications, and the interplay of them all until the facts are laid out in logical order in the descriptive and analytic narrative. Putting things on paper gives a perspective of what you know compared to what you thought you knew almost better than anything else you can do.

Last, after the first or second draft has been written, wait for 10 days to 2 weeks before looking at your paper again. You will then often see your writing more objectively and critically. The evidence, the inferences, the logic, the "flow" of your paper may then appear in a very different light and may need more changes.

Guidelines

Here are several guidelines that may help you in presenting the results and in the discussion. Remember you are trying to convince and persuade people to believe you.

1. Develop your findings logically. Write from the general to the specific; do not start with the minutiae and then try to encompass the whole world afterward. In the results section, try to grasp and explain the full extent of the findings at the beginning. Then focus on the individual elements one by one. In the discussion, start with the big picture, to provide an overall context or consideration, and then fix attention upon the more specific aspects of your study. If the subject is influenza in the United States or about cancer of a particular type, write several sentences about influenza or cancer in general that orient the reader, so that all the subsequent facts and findings will fit into a more understandable context. In other words, concentrate on the unfolding of facts and transition in thought.

2. Consider "friendly persuasion" in the discussion. Do not hit your reader over the head with the material that is hardest to understand or even the best evidence at the beginning. Start with simple, understandable, and accepted statements. Present the weakest supporting evidence at the beginning, then slowly build to the strongest and most plausible explanation at the end. Let your sentences grow in complexity, all the while recognizing other possible explanations as you slowly present your case. Leave the really controversial aspects to the end of the discussion—you do not want to divert the readers' attention away from the conclusions you want them to accept.

3. Develop your thesis with an overall pathogenesis in mind. That is, when you elaborate on the factors that putatively contributed to the disease or health problem, consider the attributes of the inciting agent, the development of symptoms and signs, and the full-blown clinical presentations. How do they square with, support, and advance your presentation of the epidemiologic findings?

4. Keep your style as simple as possible. Use short words (which are usually Anglo-Saxon in derivation), short sentences, and straightforward constructions. Use the active voice when possible. It is easier to understand and is more forceful. Select words that denote rather than connote: you are an epidemiologist, not a poet.

5. Use plenty of transitional devices. Transitions are extremely important in any kind of writing. They prepare or cue the reader for a further elaboration, a change in thinking, an exception, or an unusual observation. Additionally, transitions can create a time frame that helps move the action in a desired direction. Ideally, your exposition will have transitions in thought, but if it does not, at least transitional words will help. Subheadings also cue the reader to what is to come, including the size and complexity of the subject's component parts.

Problems

Here are a few problem areas to avoid:

1. Being wrong. One of the easiest ways to "turn readers off" is to be wrong. If you state the wrong percentage or the wrong bibliographic reference or your

numbers do not add up correctly, the reader may discount everything else you say. You have then lost the battle of communicating, of convincing.

2. "Talking down" to the reader. Declarative, unmodified statements, such as "all malaria is caused by mosquitoes," often invite error and make most readers angry. The use of long and highly technical words may seemingly command power and persuade, but seldom do these expressions, per se, convince scientifically experienced and critical audiences. More often, such words confuse rather than clarify, and their frequent use suggests a kind of professional insecurity.

3. Mixing opinion with fact. One may frequently see a statement or even a phrase stating a conclusion before all the evidence is presented. This most often happens when the author states the incubation period of the disease in question before the exposure has been established. Those inferences and opinions belong in the discussion after all the facts have been presented.

PRESENTING A SCIENTIFIC PAPER

Advance Preparation

The audience

Before preparing a scientific paper, you should know something about your audience. For the lay public, students, or scientists, you will necessarily select a special format of presentation, a vocabulary, appropriate audiovisuals, and perhaps even a demeanor or style of presentation. This means that you need to think carefully of how to communicate best—how to serve the needs and desires of that audience.

The facilities

How large is the auditorium? How is it lighted? How many does it seat? How many will be there? Who controls the lights and the projector? What kind of microphone will be used? Is there a lectern, a chalkboard, a flipchart? Do you have choices about any of this? How far will you be from the first row of the audience, and how good are the acoustics? Sometimes the acoustics with a microphone are so bad that you are best understood by raising your voice unaided. Try to get answers to these questions as soon as possible. At scientific meetings, at least, try to attend several sessions in the same room a few hours in advance.

Slides versus transparencies

The first rule of thumb is not to mix slides and transparencies if you can possibly avoid it. This is confusing, wastes time, and is subject to easy error by you and/or the projectionist.

Slides require a dark room. They are generally quicker to change. One can show the "real thing"—that is, pictures of patients, places, and things. But slides are sometimes hard to make quickly and at the last minute. Equipment failures are common and can be absolutely devastating at an important scientific meeting or formal presentation. Parenthetically, it would be very smart to be sure, before you give your talk, that there are extra bulbs available for immediate replacement. With slides, you will frequently lose significant eye contact with your audience.

Transparencies are very easy to make at the last minute. They tend to promote good eye contact with the audience, particularly if you point at the transparency (not the screen) as you speak. However, they are often awkward to use because they collect static electricity and make noise, and there often is no logical place to put them when you are through. Moreover, unless you look at and check each transparency, one by one, as you show them, you can easily not center them correctly on the screen. For some, using transparencies gives the impression of teaching rather than lecturing or giving a scientific presentation. On the other hand, one can use transparencies for that delicate mixture of teaching and presenting because you can write on a transparency as you progress through your talk, underline or circle, and emphasize certain points.

In some situations, handouts can be very useful. They are particularly good for teaching and leaving your audience with the most important points you want to make, giving, in truth, a "take-home" lesson. They are ideal to use when, at the end of a field investigation, you are summarizing your findings to the local health officers. They are clearly very useful when you are concerned about electrical supply or the real possibility of equipment failure. Unfortunately, handouts have to be reproduced, they are noisy, the audience's attention is not on you but on the paper, and you lose control over them. Last, they really are not that frequently used at major scientific meetings.

The choice of slides, transparencies, and/or handouts is a personal thing. A knowledge of the setting and the formality of your talk, the nature of your audience, and the ultimate purpose of your presentation will be the best guide for deciding what audiovisual devices to use.[4]

To read or not to read

Another serious consideration is whether to read or not to read your presentation. Ideally, you will probably communicate best if you do not have to read your paper or talk. However, it usually requires years of practice, innate ability to extemporize, and a great deal of self-confidence to communicate scientific material effectively without reading it.

Again, the circumstances surrounding your talk will often dictate whether reading is essential, important, or inconsequential. Formal, major scientific presentations or guest lectureships will more likely than not necessitate reading a substantial part of your paper. This is particularly true if you are new at the game and not experienced in presenting scientific material. It is also true if there is a major time constraint (and there usually is). At most scientific meetings, one is given 10, maybe 15 minutes at most for presentations, and it is absolutely critical not to exceed your allotted time. This can best be accomplished by writing out the presentation and rehearsing it so that you are within 10 to 20 seconds of your allotted time. And, indeed, practice your talk—perhaps present it to a few colleagues or even your spouse. Get their reaction and input; it is well worth the time.

The size of the audience can sometimes help you decide whether to read or extemporize. Small audiences of up to 30 persons usually permit an informal atmosphere where your presentation can be done ad lib. When the audience comprises 50 or more, again depending upon a variety of circumstances, you may still be able to ad lib your presentation and refer frequently to notes to jog your memory. Scientific presentations to 75 or more persons probably dictate a formal, airtight presentation that is best read, unless you are a real professional. It is the rare professional who can present a paper ad lib at a scientific meeting in exactly 10 minutes in first-rate, smooth, and clear fashion. The vast majority of presenters read their papers; with enthusiasm, knowledge of the subject, good projection of words, and modest eye contact, they can communicate extremely well to the audience.

The rule of thumb: when in doubt, read it out loud. If you rehearse and are enthusiastic, articulate, knowledgeable, and coherent, you should have little difficulty in communicating by informing and convincing.

The Actual Presentation

When called upon to give your talk, walk briskly to the lectern. There is nothing more disappointing than seeing a lecturer or presenter saunter casually up to the stage. It gives the impression of not caring, of not being prepared. Get comfortable before you start talking. Make sure the microphone is exactly where you want it. Get your visuals, your notes, your glass of water, your position behind the lectern exactly the way your want them before you start. Frequently you may need to acknowledge the person who introduced you with thanks or perhaps a joke. More often, at a true scientific meeting, there will be no introduction, but it is usually good manners to acknowledge the moderator. Listen to a few talks before your own so that you will know what manners are expected and appropriate.

Position yourself close to your slides or your transparencies so that you do not have to walk halfway across the stage to point out something or find it yourself. Usually this is no problem. Minimize walking around a great deal on the stage unless you are really in a teaching mode and/or you are going to create a dialogue with your audience. Make eye contact with your audience as frequently as possible, not contact with the microphone, the screen, or the papers you are reading from. Look about the audience, not at one place or one person. This brings them closer to you as you are talking. If there is a pointer or electric arrow, keep it as still as possible and turn it off when you are not actively pointing out something. Speak slowly and clearly. The adrenalin circulating through you while you make your presentation will almost always make your words come out faster. Speak distinctly and try to project the words to the back of the auditorium.

It usually takes about 2 minutes to read one page of double-spaced text reasonably slowly and clearly. This means that if you have a 10-minute talk, your paper should be no longer than 4 1/2 to 5 1/2 pages at the very most. Regarding projections, recall that it takes varying lengths of time to get the projectionist's attention, turn off and on the lights, and show the material. Many presenters read their paper at the same time as they show slides. However, quite often speakers ad lib when the slides appear. This adds time to the presentation—about 5 to 15 seconds per slide, because it takes the audience at least that long to digest the material.

Do not hesitate to bring in props, or the real things that you used or found in your investigation. A can of tainted food or pesticide or a piece of equipment that was associated with disease is very convincing, can be very useful, and "lightens" your presentation.[5]

Content

A 10-minute presentation will include most of the key components of a scientific article. There will often be acknowledgments at the beginning and then a brief introduction, with a statement of background and purpose. Your materials and methods must emphasize the most important parts of your investigation or analysis. You cannot go into detail here—simply state the barest essentials so your audience will know exactly what you did. Avoid referring to methods that you do not have time to explain (i.e., there should be no "black box").

State the most important results, recalling that you cannot tell the audience everything you found. This will be the longest part of your presentation. This is where you may use tables, figures, and charts, which, if well used, will generally increase comprehension and minimize explanation. Discussion comes next when, as in a written paper, you highlight what was most important, how it fits in with what is presently known, and your interpretation of the findings. Then state your conclusion—a very brief summary and what it all means, including control and prevention if appropriate.

When you are finished, say "Thank you." Do not simply stop talking at the end of your presentation. The audience does not know what to expect. Also, it is simple courtesy to thank them for listening to you.

How to Alienate Your Audience

There are some relatively simple rules which, if broken, can seriously impair your ability to communicate with your audience and at the same time make you lose credibility and/or stature.

Probably the greatest offense is taking more time than you are allotted. This is selfish, it is unfair, and, if there is a discussion period set aside for your paper, you are using time that is not yours. The discussion is time for the audience to react to your presentation. Exceeding your time will infuriate most moderators, and, this is a gross abuse, you stand to suffer the major embarrassment of being asked to stop talking and to sit down. Furthermore, taking more time than allowed implies that you were not well prepared and did not know what the important points to make were. All of which boils down to the simple fact that you must not and cannot expect to present everything you did or found. You must be selective. Perhaps part of the discussion can touch on some areas that you could not present during your allotted time.

The next major problem concerns slides and transparencies. You are responsible for the quality and order of your projections. If they are out of order or upside-down or illegible, this will materially detract from your ability as a communicator and even your credibility as an epidemiologist. For some strange reason, some people simply do not care about their visual aids. They seem to be above it all. Do not be one of them. If at all possible, bring your own slide carousel and put your slides in the carousel yourself. Check them at least two times before you make your presentation. Nothing can ruin a first-rate presentation faster than an upside-down or backwards slide or transparency. Do not use projections that are illegible or have too much data on them. This can easily be avoided simply by projecting the slides or transparencies in a room roughly the size of the room where the meeting is. If you cannot read them easily at the back of the room, you have no business wasting everyone's time showing them.

Do not talk down to the audience. This is hard to define easily, but avoid pompous attitudes, long words, or an air of superiority. Along the same line, remember that the moderator is your supervisor; do not disregard his or her requests. It can cause great embarrassment and loss of credibility if you do not follow the moderator's instructions.

Do not become angry or upset in front of your audience. This is especially a hazard during the discussion periods. Compliment the questioner on his or her question; stay composed; say you don't know if you don't know; respect the opinions of others even if they are outrageous; and remain calm and pleasant even if you are furious underneath.

In sum: Whether you are writing or speaking, your primary purpose is to transfer facts and ideas so your audience will understand and believe you. Keep your words simple, your logic clear and understandable, and your tone one of friendly persuasion. And always remember, don't tell your audience everything you did.

REFERENCES

1. King, L. S. (1991). *Why not say it clearly: A guide to expository writing.* (2nd ed). Little, Brown and Company, Boston.
2. Huth, E. J. (1987). *Medical style and format: An international manual for authors, editors, and publishers.* ISI Press, Philadelphia.
3. Berkelman, R. L., Martin, D., Graham, D. R., et al. (1982). Streptococcal wound infections caused by a vaginal carrier. *Journal of the American Medical Association,* 248, 2680–82.
4. Mandel, S. (1987). *Effective presentation skills: A practical guide for better speaking.* Crisp Publications, Inc., Los Altos, California.
5. Heinich, R., Molenda, M., Russell J. D. (eds.). *Instructional media and the new technologies of instruction* (4th ed), pp. 54–57. Macmillan Publishing Co., New York.

11

SURVEYS AND SAMPLING

J. Virgil Peavy

This chapter deals with the essentials of survey and sampling design that can be used in the field. Simple concepts and practices are discussed. More complex methods for use in special situations are described in more advanced texts, but the tools and methods discussed below should serve well in most field investigations.[1-5]

PURPOSE OF SURVEYS

Surveys are done when there is a question to be answered and there is no existing data source to provide the needed information. A survey is a lot of work and should never be conducted when the information can be obtained more readily elsewhere. For example, one would never want to collect survey data that can be routinely obtained from a Census Bureau publication or from some other source. So it is necessary to define clearly the purpose for a survey.

TYPES OF SURVEYS

Surveys can be classified in a number of ways. One distinction is between a census or complete survey (in which every element in the target population is included) and a sample survey (in which only a portion of the target population is selected). Most health-related surveys are sample surveys.

Surveys can also be classified by their method of data collection. There are mail surveys, telephone surveys, personal interview surveys, and observational surveys. There are also newer methods of data collection by which information is recorded directly into computers. These include measurement of the television audiences carried out by devices attached to a sample of TV sets that automatically record into a computer the channels being watched.

Mail surveys are seldom used to collect information from the general public because names and addresses usually are not available and the response rate tends to be low. However, the method may be highly effective with members of particular groups, such as subscribers to a specialized magazine or members of a professional association. For field studies, mail surveys are slow and usually not representative. Telephone interviewing is an efficient method of collecting some types of data and has become quite popular in the United States. Investigations of epidemics frequently rely on telephone surveys because they are quick, inexpensive, and sensitive (i.e., they quickly reveal whether a problem truly exists). Unfortunately, cooperation with telephone surveys by the public has recently begun to decline, particularly in large cities. Also, populations with and without telephones may differ, creating a possible important bias.

A personal interview in a respondent's home or office is much more expensive than a telephone survey, but it is necessary when complex information is to be collected. Some information, such as the characteristics of the respondent's home, may be best obtained by observation rather than questioning.

Many surveys combine these various methods. Survey workers may use the telephone to "screen" for eligible respondents and then make appointments for personal interviews. Sometimes survey data are also obtained with self-administered questionnaires filled out by respondents who are members of certain groups (e.g., a group of people who attended a large dinner that is being investigated because of possible food-borne illness).

DEFINITION OF SAMPLING

Sampling is a procedure by which a specified number of persons in a population is selected for study with the hope that they are representative of the entire population. The observations, measurements, and analyses of these members allow one to draw conclusions regarding the entire population. Therefore, sampling is not merely the selection and investigation of some members of a population as a substitute for all members. Rather, it involves the use of probability theory to gain a demonstrable degree of reliability and to do so at minimal cost.

ADVANTAGES OF SAMPLING

Sampling is a method of gathering information that is otherwise impossible to obtain. Seldom do public health budgets have the resources for large-scale surveys. Therefore, sampling methods are used, for example, to monitor food and drug quality, water quality, and many other elements of public health.

The main advantage of sampling is that it permits the gathering of certain facts about a large population relatively quickly and cheaply. Furthermore, proper sampling techniques provide a measure of the amount of error inherently introduced by the sampling process. Any estimate made from a sample is subject to error, but sampling errors have the favorable characteristics of being controllable through the size and design of the sample. Sampling errors, even for small samples, are often the least of the errors present. (See below for a listing of other sources of error.)

Well-designed sampling will usually provide more accurate information than a census-based study. A few reliable, well-trained investigators working on a properly selected sample of the population can usually obtain information more accurately than would be possible for a larger team of field staff who were less well trained interviewing all individuals of a population. With available resources concentrated on a sample of a large population, the increase in sampling error from surveying a smaller number of persons will be more than compensated for by the reduction of other sources of error.

CRITERIA FOR A GOOD SAMPLING PLAN

Naturally, one will want to achieve the highest degree of reliability for the resources available. And reliability is determined by accuracy and completeness.

First, specify the amount of sampling error that can be accepted. Be sure to design the sample in such a way that one can later compute the sampling error. Recall that the sampling error varies by the size and design of the sample.

Next, consider the character and magnitude of other possible errors from other sources and make allowances for them. Some of them include the following:

- Failure to state the problem carefully and to decide just what statistical information is needed.
- Failure to define the population about which you want information with sufficient precision.
- Errors in response, voluntary and involuntary, due to misunderstanding, misinformation, misrepresentation, faulty memory, etc.
- Bias in response arising from the interviewer.

- Imperfections in the design of the questionnaire and tabulations of the results.
- Bias arising from nonresponse (i.e., the bias from the fact that answers were not obtained from all in the sample and from the fact that these nonrespondents differ from the respondents in the characteristics being measured).
- Bias arising from an unrepresentative date of the survey or of the period covered.
- Processing errors (coding, editing, calculating, tabulating, tallying, posting, and consolidating).

Last, the field aspects of a survey are most important and should be taken into consideration at every stage of the survey design. This means that the sample design should be practical, yet sample theory and practice should be compatible.

DETERMINING THE SAMPLE SIZE

Ideally, the sample size chosen for a survey should be based on how reliable the final estimates must be. In practice, usually a trade-off is made between the ideal sample size and the expected cost of the survey. The size of the sample must be sufficient to accomplish the purpose but should not be more than necessary, or it becomes wasteful. The following items determine the sample size:

- The confidence level and precision desired.
- The variability of the characteristics being measured in the target population. If unknown, you must assume maximum variability.
- The size of the target population.

The most common method of sampling is to determine what proportion of a population has some characteristic (e.g., immunized, hypertension, exposure to a toxin). When sampling to estimate a proportion, the following formula is used in the determination of sample size:

$$n = \frac{t^2 pq}{d^2}$$

where n = first estimate of sample size
     t = confidence (for 95%, use 1.96)
     d = precision (0.05 or 0.10 usually)
     p = proportion in the target population with the characteristics being measured (if proportion is unknown, let p = 0.5).
     q = 1–p

Once n is calculated, compare n with the size of the target population (N). If n is less than 10 percent of N, then use n as the final sample size. However, if n is greater than 10 percent of N, then use the following formula to adjust for a small target population:

$$n_f = \frac{n}{1 + \dfrac{n}{N}}$$

where

n_f = final sample size
N = size of target population

Then n_f must be appraised to see whether it is consistent with the resources available to take the sample. This demands an estimation of the cost, labor, time, and materials required to obtain the proposed sample size. It sometimes becomes apparent that n_f has to be drastically reduced. If this happens, you are faced with a hard decision: whether to proceed with a much smaller sample size, thus reducing precision, or to abandon efforts until more resources can be found.

BASIC TYPES OF SAMPLES

Probability sampling is the use of statistical theory in the design of a field investigation when sampling will be done. This type of sampling is unbiased and enables you to draw valid conclusions about the population from which your sample was drawn. It is the selection of a sample such that every member in the population has a known and nonzero probability of being included.

Subjective (judgment) sampling is the selection of a sample based on someone's judgment and knowledge of the subject matter. This type of sampling is biased and generally used only when there is not time to define a probability sample. An example might be a quick sampling of children's immunization status following a natural disaster, based on recollections of local health care professionals.

Convenient (chunk) sampling is the use of a sample that is near at hand and is inherently biased. Route samples, streetcorner political surveys, or a sample based on persons coming to a clinic are convenient samples.

PROBABILITY METHODS USED IN SELECTING SAMPLES

Simple random sampling gives every member of the population an equal chance of being included in the sample. It requires a listing of every member of the population. A table of random numbers may then be used to select individuals for the sample. Simple random sampling is theoretically simple but often unrealistic in practice because it can be expensive and may present difficulties such as geographic dispersion of the study population.

Since no control of the distribution of the sample is exercised in this case, some samples may be poorly distributed (not biased, but unrepresentative). Therefore, simple random sampling is usually not desirable, though certain variations and improvements can be made to increase the accuracy of the sample. The principle of simple random sampling is the basis of all good sampling techniques and can be utilized in each of the following more specialized techniques.

Systematic sampling is often used when elements (e.g., individuals) can be ordered or listed in some manner. Rather than selecting all subjects randomly, one determines a selection interval, picks a random starting point, and selects every nth person (the same as a selection interval) on the list. Good geographic distribution (according to population density) can be assured. It is an easy method to apply and a popular one among public health professionals.

In stratified sampling, the target population is divided into suitable, non-overlapping subpopulations or strata. Each stratum should be homogeneous within and heterogeneous between other strata. A random sample is then selected within each stratum. Each stratum is more accurately represented, and since members are more alike within each stratum, the overall sampling error is reduced. Separate estimates can be obtained from each stratum and an overall estimate can be obtained for the entire population defined by the strata. This method is used frequently in immunization surveys, animal surveys, and environmental surveys.

Cluster sampling is of particular value to save resources in surveys of human populations when the population is geographically dispersed. In this type of sampling, the units sampled first are not the individual elements in which we are ultimately interested but rather clusters or aggregates of those elements. For example, in sampling the population of a rural area, a sample of villages may be selected and some portion or all of the households in the sample villages may then be included in the sample. It is apparent that such a sample involves less traveling than a simple random sample of households of the same size. This type of sampling almost always loses some degree of precision. To maintain the same degree of precision as in simple random sampling, one would have to approximately double the sample size.

Multistage sampling involves sampling of different levels of population groupings. It is used in large-scale surveys where a list of the final sample units would be too large. Selecting housing units in a large metropolitan area would usually be accomplished with two to four stages. Consider, for example, a survey of smoking habits of junior high school and high school students in a county. We could designate the first stage, or primary sampling units, as the schools in the county. The second stage, or secondary sampling units, are the home rooms within the schools. The tertiary sampling units are the individual students within the home rooms. To select the sample, list the schools and select some. For each sampled school, make a list of home rooms and select some. For each sampled home room, make a list of students and select some. An obvious advantage here is that you only need a listing of the students in the selected classrooms.

Multiphase sampling is used to obtain supplementary information. Certain information is taken from a sample while additional information is taken from a subsample. For example, an immunization survey is designed and the data are to be analyzed by socioeconomic areas (high, middle, low) and nursing districts where the districts overlap socioeconomic boundaries. These surveys can be very complex and very difficult to design and implement.

Area sampling is a geographic grid system method frequently used for environmental surveys that determine rat infestation, mosquito counts, and similar problems. Population density is usually not taken into consideration as the grid is drawn over a map. However, in some instances, the size of the grid may require adjustment, particularly for very high or low population densities.

MATERIALS NECESSARY FOR SURVEY DESIGN

Survey materials must be prepared and issued to each interviewer, including ample copies of the questionnaire; a reference manual; information about the identification and location of the sample units; and any cards, pictures, or letters to be shown to the respondents. However, these items are normally developed after the survey design. The specific materials needed to determine sample size and to select the sample are as follows:

- Maps of all survey areas with clearly defined streets, business districts, parks and cemeteries, areas of no housing, and other details that may be desired.
- Data from the most recent census to yield information on education, income, housing, age distribution of the population, number of persons per household, and other data needed to determine the sample size and to select the sample.
- Good knowledge of any changes that have taken place since the last census. It is often necessary to adjust your design slightly to eliminate field problems later.

Many of these needed items may not be available and may have to be obtained by preliminary field work. For example, housing counts on blocks may have to be done before the sample can be selected.

DEVELOPING AN INTERVIEW FORM

Good epidemiologists do not collect data, determine how to analyze the data, and then see if these analyses solve the problems they have posed. Instead, the problem and the appropriate analysis of the data determine what should be collected and how. The first step in a study using a questionnaire is not devising the questionnaire itself; that is the last step. Your first step is to state the problem in such a way that it can be solved. The appropriate analysis that will solve the problem must then be selected. This, in turn, will determine the kinds of tables that you will make. It is important to construct table shells before the data are collected (see Chapters 7 and 8). The methods for collecting the data to fill in these tables are then predetermined. Once this process is completed, consider the following few general rules and comments for questionnaire design:

- It should be as simple as possible and easy to code.
- It should have a few lead questions that will put the interviewee at ease.
- It should collect the needed information and not be too lengthy.

Two types of questions are frequently used:

1. Multiple-choice. Several different answers are given and only one is acceptable. "True-false" and "matching" are variations.
2. Open-end or free-answer. The answer is written by the respondent. "Fill in the blank" or "complete the sentence" are variations of this type. Recall that frequently, particularly in large surveys, analyses of answers of open-ended questions can be very time-consuming. Moreover, the responses may be hard to categorize and their interpretation very subjective.

GETTING ACCURATE INFORMATION

The interviewer must always be aware that errors in response—both voluntary and involuntary, due to misunderstanding, misinformation, misrepresentation, faulty memory, and the like—can and will occur. To help get accurate information from an interviewee, several things should be done, if possible:

- Conduct a training session for interviewers that stresses such issues as how to make initial contacts and how to avoid influencing or biasing responses.
- Collect information by means of standardized questions so that every individual surveyed responds to exactly the same question.

- Field test the interview form to ensure that interviewees will understand the questions. Local terminology must be used. Painful or embarrassing questions should be eliminated.
- Where possible, assure the interviewee that all information given is confidential and will be mass-tabulated (see Chapter 14). When appropriate, the interview forms should be destroyed after tabulation, and the names and addresses of survey respondents should be safeguarded.
- Periodically analyze the results to keep a check on accuracy. You can include known elements in the survey or select a sample of unknown elements for verification. For example, in an immunization survey, you could include some families whose exact records are known (not to be tabulated with the survey population) and then compare those records with what they tell you during the interview. The other method is to randomly select some families from the survey population, determine their true records, and then compare the data with what they said.
- Randomize field assignments to minimize interviewer bias. For example, do not allow interviewers to remain in the same socioeconomic strata for an extended time period.

SHORTCUTS TO AVOID

Conducting a creditable survey entails scores of activities, each of which must be carefully planned and controlled. Taking shortcuts can invalidate the results and badly mislead you. Four of the shortcuts that occur too often are as follows:

- Failure to use probability sampling procedures. One way to ruin an otherwise well-conceived survey is to use a convenience sample rather than one based on probability design. It may be simple and cheap, for example, to select a sample of patients attending a public clinic in order to get some needed information. However, this sampling procedure could give incorrect results, since these persons are unlikely to be representative of the entire community.
- Failure to pretest to the field procedures. A pretest of the questionnaire and field procedures is the only way to find out if everything "works," especially if the survey employs a new procedure or a new set of questions. It is rarely possible to foresee all the possible misunderstandings or bias effects of different questions and procedures. The pretest is usually a small-scale pilot study to test the feasibility of the intended techniques or to perfect the questionnaire concepts and wording.

- Failure to follow up nonrespondents. It is not uncommon for the initial response rate of a survey to be under 50 percent. Your plan must include returning to sample households where no one was home; persuading persons to participate who are inclined to refuse; and, in the case of mail surveys, contacting all or a subsample of the nonrespondents by telephone or personal visit to obtain a completed questionnaire. A low response rate does more damage in rendering a survey's results questionable than a small sample alone, since there is no valid way of scientifically inferring the characteristics of the nonrespondent population.
- Failure to use adequate quality control procedures. You should check the different facets of a survey at all stages—checking sample selection, verifying interviews, and overseeing the editing and coding of the responses, among other things. Without proper quality control, errors can occur with disastrous results, such as selecting or visiting the wrong household, failing to ask questions properly, or recording the incorrect answer. Insisting on proper standards in recruitment and training of interviewers helps a great deal, but equally important is proper review, verification, and evaluation to ensure that the execution of the survey corresponds to its design.

PLANNING AND IMPLEMENTING A SAMPLE SURVEY

A survey usually has its beginnings when you, the field epidemiologist, are confronted with an information need and there are no existing data that suffice. You should take the following steps in planning and implementing a sample survey:

- Lay out the objectives of the investigation. The problem must be stated in such a way that it can be solved. The objectives should be as specific, clear-cut, and unambiguous as possible. For example, the objective of a survey may be to estimate the prevalence of smoking among 12- to 18-year-olds or to determine the food histories of all persons attending a banquet.
- Define and locate the target population. There should be a clear statement of who represents the target population and where they are located geographically.
- Determine what resources are available. The number of people (and their backgrounds); amount of funding; availability of computers, telephones, motor vehicles; and the time constraints for completing the study all will have profound effects on the design, conduct, and analysis of the survey.
- Determine the sample size. The required accuracy level of the data has a direct bearing on the overall survey design. You can estimate the approxi-

mate number of persons to be sampled mathematically when you know the amount of sampling error that can be tolerated in the survey results and the particular sampling method to be used.

- Determine the sampling method to be used and select the sample. It is most important to take into consideration the field aspects of the survey during this phase. Whatever you design in advance must have easy application in the field. Usually, the sample can be selected in two or three stages, with some of the random selection being done by the interviewers.
- Decide on the mode of data collection. The mode—personal interview, telephone interview, or mail—must be appropriate for the objectives, resources, and target population.
- Decide how the data will be processed/analyzed. Good data management should be part of the survey design. Will the data be collected on questionnaires, on answer sheets, or directly into a personal computer? How and by whom will the questionnaires be processed and stored? Does the sampling method require special analytic techniques to take the design effect into account?
- Develop, field test, and revise the questionnaire. Designing the questionnaire is one of the most critical stages in developing a survey. The questionnaire links the information need to the actual measurement. Unless you define the concepts clearly and the questions unambiguously, the resulting data are apt to contain serious biases.
- Train the interviewers and conduct the fieldwork. Survey-control measures are most important during this stage. They include the need to collect data systematically and to select each respondent in each sample unit properly. Remember that a key part of the fieldwork is dealing with nonrespondents. There must be a systematic plan for revisits, telephone calls, or other follow-up to increase the completion rate.
- Check all interview forms for coding errors. It is usually necessary to have a well-trained person carefully check for coding errors. Do not allow interviewers to check for their own errors.
- Enter, tabulate, and analyze the results. This phase can usually be accomplished with a personal computer. However, remember that you can lose data when electricity fails (not uncommon in overseas investigations), with disastrous results. Back up the data on a floppy disk at regular intervals, and save the questionnaires until you are certain they are no longer needed.

The analysis of survey data may require specific techniques to account for the sampling method used. *SUDAAN* (Survey data analysis) and other software packages are now available to analyze complex survey data on the personal computer. Begin with the descriptive epidemiology so as to become familiar with the data and to ensure that the data appear to be representative. Then proceed to more complex analyses as necessary. In interpreting the data, recognize the limitations of the design, conduct, and analysis of your survey.

REPORT THE RESULTS

As in all epidemiologic work, the survey should be described in a written report (see Chapter 10). The report should include the survey's objectives, methods, results, your interpretation of the findings, and your conclusions. The report serves not only as documentation of the work that has gone into the survey but also as a means of communication to decision makers, such as policymakers, funding sources, and program managers.

REFERENCES

1. Cochran, W. G. (1953). *Sampling techniques*. John Wiley and Sons, Inc., New York.
2. Levy, P. S., Lemeshow, S. (1980). *Sampling for health professionals*. Lifetime Learning Publications, Belmont, California.
3. Abramson, J. H. (1974). *Survey methods in community medicine*. Churchill Livingstone, Edinburgh and London.
4. Barker, D. J. P. (1973). *Practical epidemiology*. Churchill Livingstone, Edinburgh and London.
5. World Health Organization (1986). *Sample size determination*. World Health Organization, Geneva.

12

USING A MICROCOMPUTER
FOR FIELD INVESTIGATIONS

Andrew G. Dean

In the past decade the microcomputer has become an important tool for epidemiologic field investigations. Epidemiologists routinely use portable computers in field investigations along with questionnaires, statistics, laboratory tests, and other more traditional epidemiologic tools.

A computer is a machine, and, like most machines, it requires an investment of technical skill and setup time that can be recovered through increased quantity and quality of output.

Computers are most useful for:

1. Tasks that are clearly defined and that will be done many times in the same way
2. Rapid computation or counting involving large numbers of similar records
3. Tasks matching the capabilities of existing software
4. Numerically intensive calculations
5. Accurate retention of details
6. Investigators who have used the same system before

Manual processing is still indicated for:

1. One-time or occasional tasks
2. Small numbers of records

3. Complex or changing tasks
4. Operators who are not familiar with computer use
5. Situations where staffing for manual tasks is easier to obtain than computers or knowledgeable operators

Tasks that may be usefully performed on a computer during an outbreak investigation include word processing, processing of questionnaire data, analysis of existing electronic data, computer communication, and bibliographic searching.

MICROCOMPUTERS

The pace of progress in the miniaturization of computers in the past 15 years has been nearly miraculous; therefore a description of microcomputer hardware is sure to be outdated as soon as it is printed. At present, a portable computer and printer can be carried to the field in a briefcase and operated either from batteries or standard electrical power. The computer may have a hard disk capable of storing thousands of questionnaire records and generally would have most of the features of its desktop cousins at the office at a slightly higher cost. Portable modems make it technically possible to send files or access remote databases from any area with telephone service, although some countries place restrictions on modem use.

The most common type of microcomputer is the IBM-compatible computer with the DOS or Microsoft Windows operating system. Since IBM-compatible microcomputers are ubiquitous and also permit fairly easy development of software, most epidemiologic software is available for these models. The Macintosh computer, known for its ease of use and minimal barriers to learning, is now available in "notebook" size models that should increase its use in the field. Both types of computers are fairly rugged and light enough to carry, and some models are easily adapted to international electrical variations. The overall issues in choosing a computer include compatibility with other computers in the home office and field environment, availability of epidemiologic and statistical software, and the usual factors of cost, capacity, speed, durability, and repair service.

SOFTWARE

The type of software available for epidemiologic investigation is of more importance than the brand of computer or operating system. During a field investigation, software may be needed for word processing, data entry, database management, data analysis and statistics, communications, bibliographic searching, and miscellaneous functions such as scheduling and note-taking.

Commercial programs are available for word processing, scheduling, note-taking, graphing, and other functions that are common business applications. Data entry and database management can be done with commercial programs such as *dBASE* and *Paradox*, but these do not offer statistics for epidemiology, and setting up databases and manipulating records requires more attention than many investigators are able to spare in a busy field situation. This software is quite expensive if multiple copies will be required.

Statistical software is available commercially, the most popular general purpose programs being *Statistical Analysis System (SAS)*[1] and *Statistical Programs for the Social Sciences (SPPS)*.[2] They both require considerable amounts of hard disk space but will perform a wide variety of statistical procedures for those familiar with the statistics and with programming in *SAS* or *SPSS*. Since their commands are different from those of the database programs, the use of both statistics and database programs requires learning two "languages." Both *SAS* and *SPSS* offer facilities for data entry and thus may be used without a database program, although data entry usually cannot be controlled to the extent that it can in a database program. Epidemiologic fieldwork often requires statistics for categorical (coded or yes/no) rather than continuous data. Mantel-Haenszel analysis of stratified data is important, and for those who know how to use and interpret it, logistic regression may be desirable after preliminary Mantel-Haenszel analysis. It is important that entry, checking, coding, and editing of data be easy to perform. Setting up a new questionnaire is almost always required in a field investigation, and this should be easy to do in the software that is chosen.

The Centers for Disease Control and Prevention and the World Health Organization have developed a program called *Epi Info*[3,4] for use in epidemiologic investigations; it attempts to provide the best compromise between ease of use and flexibility. It is in the public domain and may be copied for use by others. Versions are available in French, Spanish, Arabic, Russian, and Chinese, and translations of the manual in several other languages. In this chapter we will use *Epi Info* to illustrate many of the tasks to be performed with computers in the field. A companion program called *Epi Map*[5] provides features for producing and editing community maps in the field and for displaying epidemiologic data through shading, patterns, or dots on the map. Other free and inexpensive software for use in epidemiology is listed from time to time in the *Epidemiology Monitor*.[6]

Whatever software is chosen, it is important that the investigator be familiar with its use and limitations before leaving for the field. A tense field situation with high stakes and an insistent press leaves little time for learning about software or devising programs to solve new problems. The analysis does not have to be sophisticated, but it should be correct with regard to the totals obtained and the elementary statistics. Logistic regression can wait until later, but the basic data must return from the field intact, properly backed up, and well documented.

THE WORKING AND TRAVELING ENVIRONMENT

To minimize problems in the field, hardware, software, and operator skills should have been used as much as possible before leaving the home office. At the very least, a "dress rehearsal" should be conducted before leaving to be sure that all necessary elements are available.

Magnetic disks must be treated like fine phonograph records and protected from fingerprints, scratches, coffee, magnets, sharp bending, and denting by firm objects like ballpoint pens. They will not be harmed by a reasonable number of passes through a modern airport x-ray machine, but the metal detectors through which passengers walk do generate magnetic fields that could be harmful to diskettes. Diskettes should be protected from both heat and intense cold. They should never be left in a parked car in warm weather.

When traveling to other countries, it is important to be sure that the type of power (120 vs. 240 volts) and connecting plug are known and compatible with the equipment being used. With appropriate adapters, portable computers may be run from car batteries, or even by solar power in remote locations. Battery power is much less subject to effects from voltage variations found in many developing countries. Some countries require prior clearance for bringing a computer in or out. Others have restrictions on the use of modem communications. It is important to check on such regulations with appropriate embassies, scientific colleagues, or customs officials.

In the field, the computer work space should be shielded from direct sun and protected from dust. The power cord for the computer should be fastened to the outlet with tape or other means so that power will not be accidentally interrupted.

Organization of a portable computer's hard disk can contribute greatly to ease of use. Some investigators recommend creating a new directory for each investigation, keeping all files pertaining to that investigation in the same directory. The profusion of disk sizes and densities, even on IBM-compatible microcomputers, can lead to problems in transferring data from one computer to another. It is useful to carry appropriate cables and software to transfer files via serial-port connections. One such product is Laplink III (Traveling Software, Bothell, WA 98011).

WORD PROCESSING

Word processing is used for producing questionnaires, plans, and reports and for recording miscellaneous observations during the investigation. A word-processing package previously used by the investigator is preferred, since considerable time may be needed to adjust to a new package.

The software (and the investigator) must be capable of producing a plain text or "ASCII" file for transfer to another word-processor. Collaborators in the investigation may use a brand of word processor with an incompatible proprietary file format, but most word processors will accept a plain text file as input.

DESIGNING A QUESTIONNAIRE FOR COMPUTER USE

A questionnaire is a tool or template for structuring data collection so that items to be tabulated by computer or by hand are all of the same type. A good questionnaire, like a computer program or written essay, begins with an outline of major topics to be addressed. Often the objective is to explore correlations between an illness or injury and one or more exposures or risk factors. The large topics in the outline would then be:

Identifiers and follow-up information
Demographic information (age, sex, etc.)
Disease
Exposures
Possible confounders

Within each section, a series of questions is identified. These are usually given names that can also serve as field or variable names in the computer file—names like FIRST NAME, SOCIAL SECURITY NUMBER, DIARRHEA, and POTATO SALAD. Each of these can be developed into a question intelligible to the subject or to the interviewer. Some, like DIARRHEA, may require several questions (ONSET DATE and TIME, FREQUENCY, CONSISTENCY, etc.) that may be summarized in a final yes/no conclusion on meeting the investigator's case definition of DIARRHEA.

In designing a questionnaire, it is useful to understand the computer program that will be used to enter and analyze the data. A few computer terms will be useful in describing data entry and analysis.

A FIELD or VARIABLE is one data item, such as FIRST NAME or AGE. Usually FIELD is used to describe the blank in which data items are entered and VARIABLE refers to the field name that may be manipulated later during analysis. A RECORD is usually the information from one questionnaire. Many records are stored together in a FILE. Files are given names of eight or fewer letters followed by a period and an optional three letters. *Epi Info* data files end in .REC, as in DATA01.REC. A file may be recalled for analysis or data entry, stored on floppy or hard disks, and copied from one disk to another.

A field usually has a textual question or prompt, a maximum number of characters (length), and a name (up to 10 characters in *Epi Info*). In *Epi Info* for example, a questionnaire (and a database specification) might be a file, created on a word processor, that begins with the following lines:

Division of Epidemiology
Public Health Department

{Id}entification {Num}ber ###
Name _____ Age ## Sex <A> (M/F)

Epi Info would automatically create four fields as follows:

Field name:	IDNUM	NAME	AGE	SEX
Field type:	Numeric	Text	Numeric	Upper-Case Text
Field length:	3	22	2	1

In *Epi Info* a pound or number symbol (#) requires numerical input. An underline allows any kind of text. The <A> represents an upper-case text field that converts entries to upper case, to avoid having sexes ("m," "M," "f," and "F") during the analysis phase, for example.

Other data entry programs may ask the user to specify "field name," "field type," and "field length" for each individual field as the database or file is being set up. The end result is the same: the program displays a prompt on the screen and allows entry of data in a blank field. Almost all data entry programs accept data of the specified type (e.g., numeric) and reject other entries (e.g., "Jones" in a numeric field). Many have sophisticated methods for evaluating entries and taking appropriate action to prevent erroneous entries. In *Epi Info*, for example, a program called *CHECK* allows specification of minima, maxima, legal codes, skip patterns, automatic coding, and copying of data from the preceding record. By inserting statements in a special check file, the user can set up more complex checks to issue an error message if a particular date precedes another date or a diagnostic code conflicts with the person's age or gender. Check files can also be set up to do mathematics or to call another program to perform complex calculations and put the results in other parts of the data entry form.

Complex checking on data entry has a cost in terms of set-up time and skill required. During an outbreak investigation with *Epi Info*, most epidemiologists would insert a few checks, such as maxima and minima or legal codes, and would tell the program to skip questions shown to be irrelevant by previous answers (e.g., skip the section on symptoms if the person was not ill). If several different people will be entering the data, it may be worth spending extra time to set up checks for consistency and acceptability; but this may not be worth the trouble if one person enters all the data and the number of records is small enough to allow manual checking after entry.

In some situations, it is preferable to enter data directly into the computer rather than using paper forms first. Direct entry has been used in door-to-door survey work and for abstracting records in medical record rooms. In most outbreak investigations, however, a paper form will be used for interviews and the results will be transferred to a computer later, perhaps in a health department office or in a motel room with a portable or laptop computer.

There are two styles of questionnaire images that may be used on the computer screen. The first is a telegraphic or "keypuncher's" form. It consists of field names and data entry blanks only, arranged on the screen to allow the fastest possible entry by a person thoroughly acquainted with both the paper and the screen forms. Such a questionnaire might begin as follows:

```
Idnum      ####
Name       _____
Age        ##
Sex        <A>
County     <A>
Disease    <Y>
Chicken    <Y>
Ham        <Y>
Beef       <Y>
```

The second style is an extended format that resembles the paper form as closely as possible, complete with headings, questions, instructions to the user, and blanks. With slight editing, the same form may be used in an actual interview. This format is most useful if there are relatively few questionnaires, there are several people entering the data who do not have time to become "experts" on the data format (entering 100 questionnaires might produce an "expert"), or those entering data will be frequently interrupted.

In *Epi Info*, either format may be used, according to the investigator's preference. With the extended form, field names may be explicitly chosen by placing curly brackets around the most significant 10 characters, as illustrated previously.

In using *Epi Info* and other programs, it is important to know how the program handles missing values before finalizing the questionnaire. *Epi Info* allows a missing value to be entered by pressing the <Enter> key to leave the field blank. Some programs (and a previous version of *Epi Info*) record missing values as zero for numeric fields. In these programs the questions must be designed so that there is no confusion between a true code or value of zero and a missing value where this distinction is important. "Zero" glasses of water consumed and "unknown" glasses of water consumed, for example, are quite different, so that a special code (often 9 or 99) should be assigned for the case of "unknown." Such codes are unnecessary in the current version of *Epi Info* (version 6), since missing data are stored as values distinct from zero.

In some investigations, particularly in research settings, it is useful to assign additional codes (for example, 8's) to distinguish answers cited as "unknown" by the subject, those considered less accurate or unknown by the interviewer, and those somehow omitted during data entry. These extra codes can complicate the analysis considerably and should only be assigned after careful thought about the format of the table that will show the results. "Somebody might ask about it later" is not sufficient reason to burden the investigation with a series of cumbersome codes unless their analysis accomplishes a specific objective. In a field investigation, it is often sufficient to use only one kind of missing value, since the modest number of cases and rough-and-ready data-collection process do not permit analysis of bias that may have arisen due to more than one type of missing data.

To provide proper analysis of many questions, codes must be assigned. Merely typing in the names of counties or diseases can result in a profusion of synonyms and misspellings that is impossible to analyze. In *Epi Info*, either numeric or text codes may be used. In producing tables during analysis, codes indicating the actual values are more useful than numeric codes, although numeric codes can be recoded to produce useful labels during analysis. Generally "Y" and "N" are less likely to produce errors in data entry than "0" and "1," and "URI" is more meaningful than "7002" for upper respiratory infection.

A key issue in setting up data entry forms involves multiple-choice questions. The question:

How many glasses of water do you drink per day (choose one)?
    0. None
    1. 1–2
    3. 3–4
    5. 5 or more
    9. Don't know
       Water #

Has five mutually exclusive answers; the entire question therefore has a single answer. A one-digit numeric field called WATER is enough to record the answer.

Another type of question is:

What symptoms have you had in the past month?
    1. Diarrhea
    2. Fever
    3. Chills

Note that all three symptoms might have been present. Each part of what looks like a single question requires a yes/no answer, and this question should be set up as follows:

What symptoms have you had in the past month?

    Diarrhea   <Y>
    Fever   <Y>
    Chills   <Y>

The same would be true of a list of foods possibly eaten at a meal. Each item is really a separate question, since the answers are not mutually exclusive.

In *Epi Info*, analysis of the two sample questions would proceed as follows. To obtain information on the number of persons having various levels of water consumption in the first style of question, the command FREQ (frequency) WATER will display the codes for each level and the number of times each code is represented.

The symptom question is more complicated, however. By asking for a frequency distribution of the variable DIARRHEA (FREQ DIARRHEA, in *Epi Info*), it is a simple matter to ascertain the number of persons with and without diarrhea. Discovering how *many* symptoms each person had takes more complex programming—complex enough so that it may be easier to add another summary question below the list of symptoms, such as "Number of symptoms #" if this is important for the analysis. The person entering data can quickly scan the paper form, count symptoms, and enter this number rather than requiring the investigator to do extra programming during the analysis stage.

The trade-off between intelligent data consolidation during data entry and having the computer do the work is evident at many points during design of computer entry forms and paper questionnaires. If you will be using both, consider simplifying as much as possible the data transferred to the computer from the paper form. Names, addresses, and other follow-up information may be omitted, and complex case definitions may be summarized with a single yes/no question. Field investigation usually results in scores or hundreds of questionnaires, rather than thousands, and the human mind and eye may be a simpler processing alternative for some kinds of questions than having a busy investigator with modest computer skills try to write a program to condense the data electronically.

In the end, the investigator must decide what to collect, how much of a completed questionnaire to process by hand, and in what form to code it for computer use. Although experience plays a major role, pilot testing can be a good substitute. With modern systems such as *Epi Info*, it is quite easy to enter data from five or six sample questionnaires (preferably from people who will not be included in the final study). These are then processed to produce a model for the final analysis, saving the program that results. This procedure will often reveal gaps, inconsistencies, or ambiguities in the questionnaire and point out questions that do not contribute to the analysis; it is almost guaranteed to improve the final questionnaire design. Before finalizing the design, each question should be examined with the additional questions hovering in the background, such as "What do I really want to know? " and "How am I going to process this field?"

DATA ENTRY AND VALIDATION

Usually paper questionnaires from the field are far from ready for analysis after data entry. They contain misspellings, synonyms, abbreviations, upper/lower case mixtures, marginal notes, and missing data. Data entry is an opportunity for partial "cleaning" of the data set. It must be done with scrupulous dedication to preventing bias—the kind that could insert data favorable to a hypothesis or eliminate items detrimental to it. Since field investigations seldom have the luxury of "blind" coders and data entry personnel, only strict and literal attention to accuracy can prevent bias.

It is a good idea to alternate case and control forms during data entry to avoid bias from the small decisions and adaptations that occur during the course of entering forms. If there is more than one data entry person, each should enter the same ratio of case to control forms.

In most data entry systems, including *Epi Info*, a cursor on the screen indicates where an entry will occur. The cursor jumps automatically from field to field. When an entry is made, the item is checked for correct type (numeric, date, etc.) and additional checks programmed into the check file are performed. If a problem is encountered, the program indicates this and waits for correction before going on to the next field. At the end of each questionnaire, the record is saved automatically or by answering an explicit question such as "Save data to disk? (Y/N)." In *Epi Info*, a power failure (or someone tripping over the power cord) will not result in loss of records already saved, although the partial record being entered may have to be reentered. If other programs do not have this feature, save the work frequently. It is a good idea to mark each paper questionnaire as data entry is completed to avoid accidental reentry.

When all records have been entered, the entries should be carefully validated to be sure that they represent the source documents accurately. One person can read the data entered aloud while the other verifies that the entries represent the source document accurately.

Further checking may be done by performing frequencies on each field. FREQ* will accomplish this in *Epi Info*. An examination of the results will often disclose outliers such as "*Gf!" that crept in during a moment of distraction. These may be edited in the data entry program before the actual analysis is begun.

Some investigators prefer to have the same set of questionnaires entered in duplicate by two different operators in separate files. The *Epi Info* program *VALIDATE* may be used to compare the two files and detect and correct any differences.

ANALYSIS OF DATA IN FIELD EPIDEMIOLOGY

Analysis of a descriptive study or survey usually begins with a simple frequency for each variable (in *Epi Info*, FREQ*). Then, for a study with two or more groups, such as cases and controls, ill and well, exposed and unexposed, you would want to compare the two groups. For categorical (coded) data, the TABLES command in *Epi Info* (e.g., TABLES* ILL) will produce cross-tabulations of each variable by illness status (Y/N), with appropriate statistics for each.

Often in a case-control or cross-sectional study, a histogram or epidemic curve is needed. In *Epi Info*, the case group would first be selected before doing the histogram (e.g., SELECT CASE = "Y"). The histogram might be performed with HISTOGRAM ONSETDATE. Continuous variables such as age or diastolic blood pressure are analyzed with the MEANS command (e.g., MEANS SBP ILL) if SBP is systolic blood pressure and ILL is case status.

In most analytic programs it is necessary to use names of variables to do analysis. Unlike algebraic notation, computer notation usually allows a descriptive name (up to 10 characters in *Epi Info*) for each field.

At this point, you will have an idea how many records are in each group and how many missing values there are for each field. If missing values are displayed, many of the tables may be three by three rather than two-by-two, and the statistics that result are not as complete as those that accompany two by two tables. Some packages allow you to suppress missing values (in *Epi Info*, SET IGNORE MISSING = ON). Repeating the analysis after giving this command will omit the missing values and focus the analysis solely on records that have data for the tables and frequencies being produced. Two-by-two tables in *Epi Info* are accompanied by chi-square tests, odds ratios, risk ratios, confidence limits, and, if indicated, Fisher exact tests.

Often one or more "significant" findings may be indicated by P values less than 0.05 or confidence limits that exclude 1.0 for odds ratios or risk ratios. Further analysis to consider confounding variables is indicated, at least for frequent confounders such as age and sex. This is done by stratifying the table of interest (say SALAD by ILL), producing a separate table for each value of the confounder. In *Epi Info*, the crude table is produced by TABLES SALAD ILL and stratification by TABLES SALAD ILL GENDER.

In the stratified results, there are separate tables (strata) for males and females. The Mantel-Haenszel summary chi-square test and P value that summarize the combined tables may be compared with the results of the crude analysis. If the odds ratios in the two or more strata are similar, interaction is not present, and a difference in the crude and Mantel-Haenszel odds ratios may be taken as an indication that GENDER was a confounder. Other potential confounders such as AGE, socioeconomic status, and so on can be evaluated similarly, either one by one or in combination (TABLES SALAD ILL GENDER SES).

Stratification does not work well for small data sets if there are many strata, and variables such as AGE may need to be recoded (grouped) to produce fewer strata. A number of examples of data manipulation, including automation of a complex case definition, are included in the *Epi Info* manual in a chapter on epidemic investigation.[4]

At this point, the analysis may be complete enough for field purposes. If confounding has been identified and eliminated through stratification and interaction has been addressed (perhaps recording the results for more than one stratum rather than the overall results, as in "For people up to the age of 18, the effect was . . . ; those over 18 did not react the same way"); the significant findings must be evaluated from a biomedical point of view and distributed to interested parties.

Graphing of important findings may be helpful in visualizing or explaining results. *Epi Info* offers the commands BAR, HISTOGRAM, PIE, SCATTER, and LINE, each followed by the name of a variable (two variables for SCATTER and several for LINE), to produce graphs.

In cases where there are several significant risk factors or several confounders, logistic regression may be helpful. For logistic regression in *SAS* or *SPSS*, the *CONVERT* program in *Epi Info* may be used to produce files for importation into these programs.

MULTLR,[7] *LOGISTIC,*[8] and *CLOGISTIC*[9] are public domain or shareware logistic regression programs for microcomputers. Exportation of files for *MULTLR* is included in Version 6 of *Epi Info*. *LOGISTIC* and *CLOGISTIC* have recently been adapted by their author so that they read *Epi Info* files directly. A list of free and inexpensive programs available for microcomputers is available.[10]

OBTAINING AND USING EXISTING COMPUTERIZED DATA

Sometimes useful computerized information already exists at the site of an investigation. Hospital computer systems may have laboratory values, diagnostic information, or operative schedules; a water treatment plant may have results of water analysis, and so on. Such files may contain more information than is relevant and may be in a variety of file formats. Selection of relevant information can be done by the person managing the data system. If you specify a time period or category of record to be selected, it may be relatively easy for the data manager to create a file containing only the desired items, perhaps with only certain fields represented.

The file format is also important. Most computerized database and statistics programs, including *Epi Info*, will accept an ASCII file in fixed-field format. This means that only the 128 standard characters are included and each line represents a different record. A field is distinguished by its position on the line and always occupies a fixed number of characters. It is important to obtain a list of the fields and their types and length.

Epi Info will analyze files in the dBASE format directly and will import files in the Lotus 1-2-3, comma-delimited, dBASE, and fixed-field ASCII formats with a program called *IMPORT*.

Whenever external files of any kind are copied, the source disk should first be checked for computer viruses with a suitable program, no matter how reputable the supplier of the data. Reference data such as telephone lists or the *Epi Info* manual may be transported as files on hard or floppy disks, so that heavier paper copies are not needed.

COMPUTER COMMUNICATIONS

A computer equipped with a modem can be used to send files of any type to another computer over the telephone system. Guidelines, library searches, memos, and even programs can be exchanged with the epidemiologist's home office. A modem can also provide access to electronic mail (E-mail) systems. Fax machines or fax boards installed in a computer may be used to communicate textual or graphic material.

Communication is sometimes difficult to set up due to the variety of protocols, telephone connections, and communications programs. If computer communication is important on an investigation, practice sessions should be conducted to work out the details before leaving for the field. A variety of telephone-jack adapters can be obtained at radio or electronic stores. Methods for obtaining technical help in a community are discussed in a later section.

OBTAINING INFORMATION FROM THE WORLD LITERATURE WHILE IN THE FIELD

Unless the investigator is a specialist in the type of problem being investigated, bibliographic searching may be of great importance. In the United States (and many other countries where it is available), the *MEDLARS* database of the National Library of Medicine is the least expensive and most comprehensive source of information. It contains references and often abstracts describing millions of articles in thousands of biomedical journals. "*GRATEFUL MED*" is a computer program[11] that allows *MEDLARs* searches from a portable computer in the field. It is necessary to open an account with the National Library of Medicine and highly advisable to practice using *GRATEFUL MED* for searching before leaving for a field investigation. Most medical libraries can also perform *MEDLARs* searches; an alternative is to locate a medical library and willing librarian to perform searches near the site of the investigation.

OBTAINING TECHNICAL ASSISTANCE
DURING A FIELD INVESTIGATION

Occasionally a computer problem arises in the field that requires more expertise than the investigator possesses. Computer breakdowns, unfamiliar file formats, access to special printers or other equipment, and difficulties with telephone connections may all require assistance. With the number of microcomputers in the United States alone estimated at 35 million,[12] technical expertise is available in most communities from a variety of sources. If calling the epidemiologist's home-base support staff does not solve a problem, a search of local health departments, technical schools, computer stores, and computer clubs may lead to a person with the necessary knowledge or piece of equipment.

COMPUTER VIRUSES AND DATA BACKUP

Just as there is little satisfaction in having written a book whose only manuscript was lost in a fire, there is little satisfaction in having gathered a great deal of data that is then lost. Therefore, proper backup of computer data is essential. Whatever can go wrong should be expected to do so—perhaps more than once. In the past few years, computer viruses have been added to the list of things that can go wrong, but they are only an additional reason for careful backup procedures, which were already necessary to protect against hard disk crashes, power outages, theft, and late-night human errors.

Computer viruses are becoming more and more prevalent. They cause a variety of problems, but the most serious destroy all data on disks used in a particular computer. They may be acquired from a source outside a previously uninfected computer, either by copying files or through communication with another system.

Commercial programs are available to detect and often remove these viruses, and one of these should be used to check all disks inserted into the computer before copying any files, processing data, or running programs. If you have brought disks of software that you will copy onto a local computer for use, be sure that the disk is write-protected (notch covered with tape for 5 1/4" disks, slider open for 3 1/2" disks) before inserting your disk in the local computer, so as to prevent your disk from becoming infected from the computer.

Portable computers are attractive to thieves, and their hard disks—like all hard disks—may "crash," making data difficult or impossible to recover. More than one floppy disk copy of all data should be made on a regular basis, and the backup disks should be carefully stored in places separate from the computer itself, to rule out the possibility of complete loss from theft, carelessness, or fire. Several well-verified disks, traveling by different routes and/or stored with different people, are the best backup system. New backups should be made at intervals, perhaps every hour or two during data entry. It is also useful to have floppy disk copies of important software in case a hard disk must be replaced in the field.

Generally, in a field investigation, it is practical to give new names to each new set of backup files, so that previous files are not written over. If anything goes wrong with a current file or disk, the previous set of files may provide a good copy of most of the data set. Although good commercial programs are available for backing up hard disks, they are usually not necessary in field investigations, since the data files are usually small. The files may simply be copied to floppy disks, maintaining several such carefully labeled disks to be used in sequence.

When things go wrong, a frequent reaction is to make the problem worse through panic. If difficulties in recovering files are experienced, first obtain technical help in diagnosing the problem. If you decide to restore files from the backup disks, be sure that the write-protect function (see previous section) is set on these disks to avoid having the backups destroyed by a virus or faulty procedure. If files have been accidentally erased on the hard disk, it is important to avoid entering further records or copying files until an attempt has been made to recover them. Programs such as *Norton Utilities*[13] can restore erased files and repair many corrupted files if they have not been written over by further manipulations.

DATA CONFIDENTIALITY AND LEGAL ISSUES

Maintaining confidentiality of data on a portable microcomputer is similar to protecting a stack of questionnaires. The best protection is through maintaining careful physical custody of any disks containing data, including, if necessary, the internal hard disk of the computer. With small data sets, files can be kept on floppy disks so that the hard disk does not contain confidential data. In many investigations, names and addresses are not needed in data files, and such data should not be entered unless it is absolutely necessary. Arbitrary identification numbers are adequate for most computerized data sets. Frequently names and other identifiers may be left with the community health department and only code-identified data transported to a more central site.

Occasionally, outbreaks lead to legal proceedings for negligence or even homicide. Records of the investigation may be subpoenaed or otherwise required for legal purposes. This and the interest of good scientific documentation make it important to keep good records of the investigation and to store them in such a way that they can be accessed by appropriate parties even if the investigator moves on to another job. Analytic programs may be written with comments explaining important steps. This also facilitates reuse of the programs in another investigation.

Computer disks should be carefully labeled, and after the investigation, stored in an organized way so that others can access the files. Paper copies of the data may be made for permanent documentation and ease of filing, since computer disks lose their magnetic data after a few years. For archival purposes, the data should be copied to new disks annually.

THE FUTURE OF COMPUTERS
IN EPIDEMIOLOGIC FIELD INVESTIGATION

Future computers for field investigation will be smaller, lighter, and more powerful. Eventually both voice and handwritten input will be practical. Medical and other records will be computerized to a greater extent, offering opportunities for capturing relevant information in detail to the investigator with the skills and tools to convert data from diverse formats. Eventually, perhaps, better programs will alleviate some of the compatibility problems between various types of software, but the competitive marketplace will ensure that other types of incompatibility arise.

Like most aspects of field investigation, computer use will continue to require ingenuity and adaptation. Those who have acquired the skills for using a portable computer, however, find that the rewards in quantity and quality of epidemiologic work accomplished make it an indispensable companion in field investigation.

NOTES

Use of trade names is for identification only and does not constitute an endorsement by the U.S. Public Health Service.

Epi Info and *Epi Map* are available without charge via the Internet computer network at address:

> ftp.cdc.gov
> /pub/epi/epiinfo
> and
> /pub/epi/epimap

Two suppliers of *Epi Info* and *Epi Map* and their printed manuals are:
> USD, Inc.
> 2075A West Park Place
> Stone Mountain, GA 30087 U.S.A.
> (404) 469-4098
> Fax (404) 469-0681

Brixton Books (North America)   Brixton Books
740 Marigny Street   P.O. Box 4398
New Orleans, LA 70117   London SW9 9xJ
USA   United Kingdom

PHN (504)944-1074
FAX (504)947-8899
gfegan@mailhost.tcs.tulane.edu

REFERENCES

1. SAS Institute, Inc. (1985). *Statistical analysis system*. SAS Institute Inc., Cary, North Carolina.
2. SPSS, Inc. (1975). *Statistical programs for the social sciences (SPSS)*. SPPS, Inc., Chicago, Illinois.
3. Dean, A. G., Dean, J. A., Burton, A. H., Dicker, R. C. (1991). Epi info: A general purpose microcomputer program for public health information systems. *American Journal of Preventive Medicine*, 7, 178–82.
4. Dean, A. G., Dean, J. A., Coulombier, D., et al. (1994). *Epi info, version 6: A word processing, database, and statistics program for epidemiology on microcomputers*. Centers for Disease Control and Prevention, Atlanta, Georgia.
5. Dean, J. A., Burton, A. H., Dean, A. G., Brendel, K. A. (1994). *Epi map: A mapping program for IBM-compatible microcomputers*. Centers for Disease Control and Prevention, Atlanta, Georgia.
6. *Epidemiology Monitor* (1994). Epidemiology Monitor, Roswell, Georgia.
7. Campos, N., Franco, E. (1989). MULTLR: A microcomputer program for multiple logistic regression by unconditional and conditional maximum likelihood methods. *American Journal of Epidemiology*, 129, 439–44.
8. Dallal, G. E. (1988). Logistic: A logistic regression program for the IBM PC. *The American Statistician*, 42, 272.
9. Dallal, G. E. (1989). cLOGISTIC: a conditional logistic program for the IBM PC. *The American Statistician*, 42, 125.
10. Sullivan, K., Foster, D.A. (1991). Epidemiologic software. *The Epidemiology Monitor*, 1–11.
11. U.S. Department of Health and Human Services. *Grateful med*. National Library of Medicine (distributors). Bethesda, Maryland
12. Hansel, S. (1994). Banks going interactive to fend off new rivals. *The New York Times*, Oct. 19, section D (column 3), 1.
13. Chambers, D. (1993). *Norton utilities*. Peter Norton Computing, Inc., Santa Monica, California.

13

DEALING WITH THE PUBLIC
AND THE MEDIA

Bruce B. Dan

Epidemiologic and public health information is of little use unless it can be communicated effectively and clearly to those who will benefit most from it—the public. In the past, people learned what little they knew about health and medicine from talking to their personal physicians. But now Americans get most of their medical information from sources other than their own doctors—newspaper articles, columns in women's magazines, celebrity diet and fitness tapes, and television. According to the 1991 Nielson Report on Television, the average American watches from 24 to 44 hours of TV each week, depending on age and gender.[1]

Medical news, whether it originally comes from journal articles, scientific meetings, or official government periodicals such as CDC's *Morbidity and Mortality Weekly Report* (*MMWR*), is first filtered through and disseminated by the mass media. Learning the structure, characteristics, strengths, and restrictions of both the electronic and print media is critical to communicating a cogent health message to the public. Moreover, within the past two decades the public has grown to expect more sophisticated information from such federal agencies such as CDC, the National Institutes of Health, and the Food and Drug Administration.[2] In their thirst for information, for example, the public expects and has grown accustomed to a rapid response from health officials during newsworthy health events, such as the legionnaires' disease outbreak in 1976, Guillain-Barré syndrome after swine flu immunization in 1976, toxic exposure from Love Canal in 1979, toxic shock syndrome in 1980, eosinophilic-myalgia syndrome in 1990, and, most notably, the burgeoning problem of acquired immunodeficiency syndrome (AIDS). On a community level, the public naturally turns to local health officials during times of uncertainty. The public's health may critically depend on the advice of medical officials (for instance, after the Mt. St. Helen's eruption), or they may just need their fears calmed (as in the almost annual occurrence of an outbreak of lice in an elementary school). Regardless, knowing how the public perceives information coming through the media, and knowing how to deliver it, can determine whether or not effective preventive measures are undertaken. What follows is a brief outline of the principles and skills involved in communicating health information to the public.

BACKGROUND

Each of the media (print, radio, television) suffers from a particular form of pressure—the deadline. Unlike almost all other enterprises, news runs under an unrelenting schedule. Dan Rather, Peter Jennings, and Tom Brokaw appear on the TV screens at exactly 6:30 p.m.—they also disappear exactly 30 minutes later. This pervasive peculiarity explains many of the quirks of the news business. Each news reporter must get his or her story into print or on the air in a short time span. News a day late is no longer news.

Although newspaper deadlines exist, they are not as tight as in radio or television. For most people it does not matter whether the morning newspaper is delivered at 3:30 a.m. or 4:00 a.m. if they are going to pick it up at 7:00 a.m., but it better not get there at 8:00 a.m. Radio news must conform to broadcast schedules much more tightly, but breaking medical news can be written rapidly if needed. Television, on the other hand, is rigidly constrained because it is a visual medium— and without pictures, there is no story. Obviously, it takes time to edit and put video images together in a logical and orderly sequence.

What these facts mean is that when reporters call about a story, they generally need it that day (not tomorrow or next week), and they may need to talk to you at that moment, not later on that day. While it is vitally important to be responsible to the news media, it is also critical to be prepared when you speak to them. We will discuss later the proper balance and timing of interviews.

It is also of vital importance to understand the interplay between reporter and news source. Each has an agenda.[3] The media are in part a journalistic exercise in the principles of the First Amendment, and they are also part of the free enterprise system (i.e., a business). But they are not in the business of public health. While it may seem that news organizations are doing a public service by communicating important health information, they do so not because of an altruistic spirit but, at the bottom line, to sell more newspapers or charge higher rates for commercials. The priorities for public health and news organizations are different. Public health officials need the media to disseminate important information; the media need medical stories to sell news. In the end, good relationships between these two diverse groups benefit the public at large.[4]

GENERAL PRINCIPLES

News reporters, like health officials, vary in their characters and backgrounds. Not surprisingly, the story reported by the political science writer for a local newspaper may differ from that of the editor of the science section of the *New York Times*, but all reporters are looking for the answers to the same six questions: Who/What/Where/When/How/Why.

It is the job of epidemiologists to have the answers ready and to present them in a clear and concise manner. But, before consenting to any interview, you should ask the same six questions! Who is going to do the interview, and from what organization? What is the subject matter to be discussed, and what questions will be asked? Where will it be done (in your office where you feel comfortable and have information at hand, or in some strange TV studio)? When will the interview take place and when will it appear (tonight's evening news or next month's *Reader's Digest*)? How will the interview be conducted (videotaped or live, one-on-one with the reporter or in a group)? And perhaps most importantly, why is it being done and why with me?

Unless you have the answers to all of these questions, you probably should not be doing the interview. There is a tendency to feel honored, important, and in the spotlight when one is asked to be quoted in a newspaper or to appear with Ted Koppel on *Nightline*, but be wary of the temptation. An overeager and ill-prepared health official does more damage than good. Additionally, one should check with local, state, or national public information personnel about any prospective interviews. Each level may have its own rules of engagement with the press. Regardless, the public relations people can give sound advice on carrying out an interview, and it is good form to let them know just what is happening. They can coordinate interviews, keep track of media attention, and prevent miscommunication with the press. The best way to prevent any misunderstanding in the interview itself is to follow four simple rules:

- Tell the truth
- Do not exaggerate
- If you make a mistake—correct it
- If you do not know, say so

If you have difficulty saying "I don't know," find some other way, such as, "That's not my specialty," or "I don't have that information right now." Do not attempt to answer a question you are not knowledgeable about. You can easily lose your credibility, but, more importantly, you may also misinform your audience.

Reporters will want to give their source of news some sort of attribution, not only to identify the source but to give an air of credibility: "Dr. John Smith, epidemic specialist in diarrheal diseases. . . ." An interview may be on the record, off the record, or in between, which is called "background." If you cannot give an interview that is on the record (meaning that everything you say or do can be used and attributed to you), you probably should not be talking to the press.

By far the most important thing to remember in giving an interview is that you are there to deliver a message and to get your point across, not to answer all the reporter's questions or to make him or her happy. It is not unusual or inappropriate for a reporter and his or her source to have different agendas. But you must have a single message to deliver. This message has been referred to as a "must air" or single overriding communication objective (SOCO). Too many people try to tell a reporter everything they know about a subject, and their basic point gets lost in the clutter. Here are some rules of thumb:

- Pick out a single cogent idea and get it across
- Get it across early (the interview may end early)
- Get your message in at least three times
- Learn to say it in an interesting way

In attempting to get a single message delivered, you will be most successful if the words you use are understandable to the greatest number of people. Avoid medical jargon. It works well in a clinical setting but not with the lay public. Learn to say it simply. For instance:

- Instead of "communicate," try "say"
- Instead of "disseminate," try "send"
- Instead of "metastasize," try "spread"

Stay away from potentially confusing words like "atypical," "subclinical," "negative test results," and "positive culture." Avoid esoteric terminology such as "relative risk," "odds ratio," "controls," and even the term "epidemiology!"

Above all, avoid the temptation to "wing it." Remember that no professional goes to a performance without a script.

Although it is unusual, there is no law against using a tape recorder yourself if a reporter is using a tape recorder during the interview. This double recording may seem bizarre, but it is sometimes used during particularly hostile or sensitive interviews. You will seldom if ever need to do this, but it shows that you are not bound by any rules.

Interviews should not be hit-or-miss affairs, but carefully planned encounters. Before you agree to do any interview, the following guidelines should be followed.

Screening

- All media contacts should first be screened by your media relations staff, or, failing that, by yourself.
- Get a clear understanding of why the reporter wants to interview you. What is the precise topic? Is it to your advantage to take part? Is it in your area of expertise or is there someone more suitable?
- Establish the reporter's deadline and how much of your time is required.

Preparation

- An ill-prepared interview serves neither the reporter's nor your interests. Getting ready for an interview is as important as doing one.
- Make it clear to the reporter that you want to confine the questions to the prearranged topic. Set a time limit for the interview.
- If possible, send fact sheets, background information, and photographs to the reporter before the interview.
- Prepare for the interview. Plan your strategy. Write out your primary public health message and practice it. Draft some colorful quotes and anecdotes that illustrate your point.

The Interview

- When the reporter arrives, reconfirm the topic and the length of the interview.
- Give him or her your business card with the correct spelling of your name and organization.
- When you are both seated, ask the reporter, "How much do you know about (the interview topic)? Now you are in control and can lay out the situation as you see it—your message.
- Briefly answer the negative or irrelevant questions and move the conversation back to your message. You can prevent "fishing expeditions" by reminding the reporter that you are prepared to be interviewed on this particular topic today. You would be glad to set up an interview on another subject another day.

- Stick to your agreed-upon time limit (you may want to have your secretary call you when the time limit has elapsed). Bring the interview to an orderly close with a summary, which should be a crisp and concise version of your message.
- Arrange a follow-up procedure so that any last-minute or verification questions can be handled.

Postinterview

- Each interview, whether for the print or broadcast media, should be an opportunity to learn and improve.
- Keep an index card for every interview, jotting down the date, the reporter's name, the subject discussed, and where it appeared. Grade yourself on the interview. Did you get the message in? Grade the reporters and file your ratings for future reference. Were these reporters knowledgeable or uninformed? Are they friends or foes?
- If you discover that you have given a reporter erroneous information, correct it immediately—even if the story has already appeared. If the reporter has misstated a fact, alert him or her so it can be corrected. If your statements have been distorted and you feel that the interview has been unfairly conducted, let the reporter know. If there is no satisfactory response, inform the reporter that the issue will be brought to the attention or his or her editor.

There are no prescribed formulas for a "correct" interview. However, there are some helpful hints in conducting yourself with each of the media. Below is listed some brief advice for each type of interview you may encounter.

Print Interview

This type of interview is probably the most common and least threatening. It usually involves a one-on-one conversation with a newspaper reporter, either in person or on the phone. Most of us are reasonably comfortable talking to another person, especially about a subject where we feel confident of our knowledge. The danger is in feeling too comfortable and saying too much. The reporter will usually tape the conversation to have exact quotes on hand, but he or she may take notes to jot down important points. If the reporter calls on the phone (and the interview has already been cleared) remember that you are not required to speak right at that moment. It is perfectly acceptable to tell the reporter that you will call him or her back in 10 minutes. Hang up, collect your thoughts, jot down some notes, get comfortable, and call back when you are ready to be interviewed.

Beware of inflections. Tongue-in-cheek remarks, a sarcastic tone, and even humor do not come across reliably in the written word, and the entire meaning may be lost to your audience. Worse, precisely the opposite meaning may come through. On the other hand, the tone of the on-the-record comments may be characterized by the reporter. That is, make a statement with a condescending tone or with a smirk, and it may be reported as such. Try to speak in even, succinct, declarative sentences, but also try to be natural and informative. The print interview is the one place where you can use exact medical terms (if you explain them), because the reader can pause, reread, and study a word or phrase. The same is not true for the electronic media.

Remember that the interview is not over when the reporter stops the recorder or puts down the pen. Any comments you make during the time spent with the reporter are on the record. The interview is over when the reporter is out of earshot.

Radio Interview

Here you must be sharply aware of inflections. The only thing the listener hears is your voice. Learn to modulate your voice in pitch, volume, and cadence. A deadpan monotone is as dreary and uninformative on the radio as it is from the podium. Use your hands and make facial gestures when expressing yourself on the radio. They will not come through to your listeners, but their effect will carry emotion and inflection to your voice. Use short, preferably monosyllabic words ("give" instead of "administer," "make" instead of "fabricate"). They are easier to pronounce and easier to understand.

Many radio interviews are carried over telephone lines. Again, do not engage in an interview either live or taped until you are ready. You are not required to carry out the interview while seated at your desk. It is permissible to stand up, walk around, or do anything else that makes you comfortable (but do not tap your fingers on the desk or chew your pencil). Talk to your interviewer as you would talk to the people you meet on the street or someone you would meet in a supermarket—simply, directly, and interestingly.

Television Interview

As with print and radio, television requires a good grasp of your information and an articulate delivery. But additionally, TV interviews call for two other vitally important factors—appearance and appeal. In particular, television has the peculiar property that it is far more important *how* you say something than what you say. This may seem heretical to some and "unprofessional" to others. But it is perhaps the most critical aspect of the television medium and one that must be understood and accepted if you have any desire to transmit information through this medium.

This unique aspect of "seeing" is what also gives television its powerful impact. But if not used properly, it results in the media manipulating the interviewer rather than the other way around. Television, in the end, does not deliver information, it conveys perceptions; it does not deliver facts, it leaves impressions. As illogical as it may seem, your appearance and demeanor carry more weight than your command of information.

Television segments usually contain only a few 15- to 20-second quotes (called sound bites) from the interviewee. This means that you must be able to relate your entire message in a very short sentence and do it in an interesting and appealing way. You must also speak in short, easily understood words, since, if the viewers misunderstand you, they do not, as with newspapers, have the ability to go back and "reread" the story. Even if what you say is technically correct, TV reporters are looking for catchy sound bites (like good one-liners). If your message is dull but you also happened to mention some other extraneous but media-grabbing statement, you can imagine what will make the air. Your job is to make your message so exciting the reporter is virtually obligated to put it on. The following, again, is a brief listing of tips to enhance your ability to get your message across on television:

- Be calm and relaxed. Television cameras and strange studio lights and microphones tend to make anyone feel uptight. Viewers will be turned off by what they perceive as stiffness and formality. This only comes with practice; there are no secrets.
- Use natural eye contact. Unless told otherwise, always look at the person to whom you are speaking. That is a natural disposition. Do not look briefly at the cameras or studio monitors, it will give you a shifty appearance.
- Dress conservatively. For men, a dark jacket and tie (a red shade is preferred) and a light-colored shirt, but try to avoid bright white. Women should wear a simple dress or business suit; stay away from large, brightly-colored prints. Reflective gold jewelry, large distractive earrings, and bizarre hairdos will take the viewers' attention away from what you are saying.
- Facial expressions should be pleasant and natural. Avoid the tendency to look numb and stiff. *Smile*! It is not only all right, it is preferred—it gives your countenance a look of warmth and friendliness.
- Your body and posture should be straight but relaxed. Even a small slump looks terrible on TV (if you feel comfortable, you probably look bad). Feel free to move naturally, and use your hands when you talk (just stay away from wild gestures, especially in front of your face). Sitting forward to-

ward your interviewer lends a sense of interest and confidence; leaning back, one of indifference and aversion.

- Speak in words of few syllables. They are less likely to be mispronounced, more likely to be understood, and you can get a lot more of them in in 15 seconds. Speak in declarative sentences. Avoid answering questions with a simple yes or no.
- Use Anglo-Saxon words. They carry emotion and add vitality to your speech. Words like "live," "die," "love," "hate," "make," "save," "get," "find." People "get sick and have heart attacks." They do not "acquire illnesses and suffer myocardial infarctions."
- Avoid trying to quote exact figures from medical journals. Do not bother letting everyone know that "53.2 percent of the case-patients taking 325 mg of aspirin daily significantly decreased their relative risk of suffering a reinfarction during the study period." It is simply "more than half the people taking an aspirin a day greatly reduced their chances of a second heart attack." Get used to using terms like "most of," "the majority," "almost all," "very few."
- Be a good listener. Nothing sounds worse than trying to answer what you thought was a preplanned question when the host is actually asking something else. Do not assume you know what the host is getting at and jump over his or her lines. Hear your host out.
- Last, project conviction and confidence. Speak to your questioner with a real sense of interest and caring. It will come across to the viewer that way as well.

EPIDEMIC MANAGEMENT

The variety of immediate problems facing the epidemiologist early in a field investigation can be daunting, and the last thing in the world the field team wants to face is the news media. But that is when the public and their information gatherers want to know the answers. Epidemiologists are loathe to rule out anything, no matter how remote, in the beginning of an investigation, but the public wants simple, direct, black-and-white answers to its questions right then, not 9 months later at a scientific meeting.

The best way to learn how to handle these problems is on-the-job training. However, it is also useful to speak to people who have "been there," such as those who visited Philadelphia during the legionnaires' disease epidemic, have gone head-to-head with tampon companies, and tried to tell 3.5 million Chicago mothers what to do when *Salmonella* was growing out of every carton of milk in the

area.[5] Every epidemic is different; every local situation will have its own pecu-
liarities; but the following may prove helpful:

- Stay away from the media. This may seem contradictory after we have emphasized the importance of communication to the public, but your number-
  one job is to assist the local health officials, not to appear on *Good Morning, America*. If you are spending a lot of time appearing on camera, you
  are not working up the problem. Designate a spokesperson. Local and state
  health agencies have a public relations person who is trained and gets paid
  to communicate. Such a specialist probably knows all the media people,
  has already established good working relationships with them, and knows
  the ins and outs of the local scene. Let the public relations people handle
  the press. They will have to do it anyway after you have gone.
- Try to have your spokesperson seek out the media first in a proactive, in-
  formational manner. It looks responsible but also lets you set the agenda
  and control events. If the media find out first, it becomes "What did you
  know, and when did you know it?"
- Establish a regular press briefing time. It establishes a routine; the media
  are not caught by surprise; and it offers you, again, the chance to make
  prepared statements and control events.
- Try to keep the technologist and other allied people behind the scenes; they
  can give potentially confusing and contradictory information to the press.
  There must be one cogent message. The press likes nothing better than
  controversy. Even something as simple as two different totals for the number of cases can give the media grist for unnerving criticism. Along that
  line, try not to get into a numbers game with the press. Refrain from "up-
  ping" the numbers every day. Even with no news, an increasing number
  becomes in itself a news story and a reason for headlines.
- Above all else, coordinate information with the local, state, and national
  officials. You will not only keep all the team players happy but will also
  avoid creating controversies—since the press likes nothing better than to
  find that the state has facts that the local health department does not have,
  and vice versa. To paraphrase the late Mayor Richard J. Daley of Chicago,
  "The field epidemiologist is not there to create disorder, the field investigator is there to preserve disorder."

PRESS CONFERENCES

The news conference increases your control in getting your message out to the
media. But in the question-and-answer period, that control can be snatched way

by an aggressive reporter. Suddenly a quiet give-and-take session can turn into a feeding frenzy. To make sure that you do not end up with a negative situation, learn to shield yourself.

- Have a spokesperson open up the news conference by introducing the participants and stating the ground rules. Handouts should be distributed at the beginning of the conference. The spokesperson should tell the assembled reporters what areas will and will not be covered and for what reasons.
- Make sure you introduce yourself when you step to the microphone. Spell your name and give your position and affiliation.
- Your first sentence should be your key message. Make it memorable and mentionable. If presented well, it should be the first sound bite carried on all networks that night.
- Keep your opening statement brief and tightly focused. If it is concise, it reduces the chances that a reporter will misunderstand, interrupt, or even walk out. Speak in headlines; save the details and documentation for the handout.
- Do not just read your statement—communicate it. Look at the audience, speak with enthusiasm or concern, gesture.
- Set some ground rules for the question-and-answer session. For example, "Now I'd like to open it up briefly for a few questions. So that everyone gets a turn, I'll take one question from each of you. I'd appreciate it if you'd raise your hand when you have a question and identify yourself."
- If no questions arise, ask yourself the first question. That might break the ice and trigger other questions.
- Do not allow yourself to be bullied. When a reporter tries to interrupt you, tell him or her nicely that you would like to finish your answer. Use your hands—signaling to one reporter that you are ready to take his or her question, while gesturing with the other hand to tell another reporter that he or she is up next.
- Summing up. When you feel that your topic has been sufficiently covered, give notice that you will take one more question. Then do precisely that. Finally, briefly restate your key point, thank the audience, and leave.

SPECIAL PROBLEMS

It is not possible to cover every twist and turn of dealing with the media, but several special situations often come up that require thinking about in advance.

- Personal opinion versus local/state policy: If asked what the official local policy is on a certain subject, you should probably refer the question to the public information officer (unless you have been given the authority to be the spokesperson—a rare instance). You should feel free, in good conscience, to give your opinions on matters of science as a physician, veterinarian, nurse, or other health personnel. But policy matters are best left to those who know the policy and can take responsibility for it. If you feel foolish telling a reporter that you do not know the policy when you feel you should know it, simply say that you would like him or her to meet with the person who can best answer that question.

- Press embargoes: Many medical journals have specific release dates, and, with them, a press embargo date, prior to which no information is supposed to be published. The purpose of this is to give all media outlets an equal chance to review of the story (for example, no one gets an edge due to the vagaries of the mail), and if everyone has the medical journal in hand when the story comes out, its health message can be disseminated in a coordinated, logical fashion. Most medical reporters will receive the journal before the release date and begin working with the story. If you are called before the embargo, simply remind the reporter of the embargo and tell him or her that you are speaking with the understanding that the story will not be published before that time. If you have any particular questions, check with the journal's editorial office.

SUMMARY

In some contrast to past decades, the American public now gets most of its medical information from the media: newspapers, magazines, radio, and television. You may be asked by the media to report and comment on your findings either during an investigation or afterward. Although your mission is to protect and maintain the public's health, the primary mission of the media is not public health but to sell their product or their time. Despite these somewhat opposite objectives, the media can and should be your ally. Learn how the media operate, and cultivate some simple practices of interviewing so that you can communicate effectively with the public.

Inform the appropriate specialists before your interview. Be prepared for the interview, know what you are going to be asked about, and know the subject. Have a message to get across and do it simply, directly, and with conviction. Tell the truth, do not be afraid to say you do not know, and do not field questions in an area that is not yours. If possible, avoid the media in the field and refer them to the local health authorities. They, rather than you, should report the results of the investigation to their constituents. They, too, should comment on health policies and issues. And, last, be sure that all levels of government have the same information. Nothing destroys confidence in our health structure more than conflicting facts.

REFERENCES

1. Schramm, W., Porter, W. E. (1982). *Men, women, messages, and the media: Understanding human communication* (2nd ed.). Harper & Row Publishers, Inc., New York.
2. Delacote, G. (1987). Communicating science to the public. In *Science and scientists: Public perception and attitudes*, pp. 41–48. John Wiley & Sons, Inc., New York.
3. Jeffres, L. W. (1986). *Mass media: Processes and effects*. Waveland Press, Prospect Heights, Illinois.
4. Kubey, R., Csikszentmihalyi, M. (1990). *Television and the quality of life: How viewing shapes everyday experiences*. Lawrence Eribaum Associates, Hillsdale, New Jersey.
5. Wilkes, M. S., Kravitz, R. L. (1992). Medical researchers and the media: Attitudes toward public dissemination of research. *Journal of the American Medical Association*, 268, 999–1008.

III

SPECIAL CONSIDERATIONS

14

LEGAL CONSIDERATIONS
IN A FIELD INVESTIGATION

Verla J. Neslund

This chapter provides an overview of the legal considerations affecting an epidemiologic field investigation. Applicable federal laws and regulations are discussed. Because of the differences in state and local laws in the various jurisdictions in which such investigations are conducted, however, the discussion of nonfederal laws and regulations is necessarily generic. The chapter covers the legal bases for investigating public health problems, gaining access, collecting data, and applying intervention strategies.

LEGAL BASIS FOR PUBLIC HEALTH INVESTIGATIONS

Federal and state governments both have inherent powers to protect the public's health. Article 1, Section 8 of the U.S. Constitution gives Congress the authority to impose taxes to "provide for the general [w]elfare of the United States" and to regulate interstate and foreign commerce. The U.S. Public Health Service (PHS) and CDC are both examples of federal agencies established under the authority of the welfare clause. Under the authority of the commerce clause of the U.S. Constitution, the federal government oversees such health-related activities as the licensure and regulation of drugs, biological products, and medical devices. Although the provisions in the U.S. Constitution are broad, the activities of the fed-

197

eral government relating to public health and welfare, nonetheless, must fit within the enumerated powers.

By contrast, the public health powers of a state are very extensive, rooted in its inherent powers to protect the peace, safety, health, and general welfare of its citizens. Unlike the federal government, the states have public health powers that are not limited to specific constitutional provisions. The state's police power includes its intrinsic right to pass laws and to take such other measures as may be necessary to protect the citizenry. In many instances, states have delegated their public health responsibilities to county or municipal governments, who likewise exercise the state's broad authority to examine, treat, and, in the case of certain contagious diseases, even to quarantine citizens in order to protect the public health. The state's public health laws include not only the established statutes of the state but also regulations, executive orders, and other directives from health authorities that may have the force of law.

The courts have consistently upheld the state's exercise of its police powers to protect the public's health. The court decision usually regarded as the seminal case in the exercise of public health police powers is *Jacobson* v. *Massachusetts*, 197 U.S. 11 (1905). In *Jacobson*, the Board of Health of the city of Cambridge, Massachusetts, had issued a regulation requiring that all citizens be vaccinated for smallpox. Mr. Jacobson was arraigned and prosecuted by law enforcement officials after he refused to be vaccinated, maintaining that the regulation violated due process because vaccination was contrary to his religious beliefs. Mr. Jacobson further argued that compulsory vaccination deprived him of the fundamental right to care for his own health. In a strongly worded opinion, the U.S. Supreme Court upheld the health board's exercise of its police power in mandating the smallpox vaccinations, providing the following rationale:

> [I]n every well-ordered society charged with the duty of conserving the safety of its members, the rights of the individual in respect of his liberty may at times, under the pressure of great danger, be subjected to such restraints, to be enforced by reasonable regulations, as the safety of the general public may demand. [197 U.S. at 29.]

The exercise of the state's police powers with respect to public health matters has limitations. The U.S. Constitution provides procedural safeguards to ensure that the exercise of these powers is not excessive and unrestrained. The Fifth Amendment prohibits the federal government from depriving—without the due process of law—any person of life, liberty, or property. The Fourteenth Amendment imposes similar due process obligations on states. Due process demands that the government use even-handed and impartial procedures in the exercise of its police power. The basic elements of such due process include notice to the person involved, a hearing or similar proceeding, and the right to representation by counsel. In addition, the exercise of the state's police power should incorporate the principle of using the least restrictive alternative that would still achieve the state's interest, particularly when the exercise involves limitations of the individual's personal liberty.

Similar to the public health activities enumerated above, the inherent powers to protect the public's health provide the general authority for laws and regulations that empower health officials to conduct epidemiologic investigations. Although cooperation of institutions and individuals in epidemiologic investigations is usually voluntary, the intervention of state or local officials is within the scope of governmental legal authority. Furthermore, the police power of the state provides the necessary authority to compel cooperation in such investigations in instances in which individuals or institutions are reluctant to grant access to certain properties, records, or individuals associated with information essential to the investigation.

GAINING ACCESS

As mentioned above, institutions and individuals generally cooperate voluntarily in epidemiologic investigations. However, if investigators meet with resistance, local or state public health officials may take legal actions, such as applying to a court with jurisdiction over the agency (individual) for a subpoena or court order to compel the agency to grant investigators access to the premises or records at issue. An individual can be compelled by court order to provide the information necessary to the public health investigation.

Institutions or individuals being investigated may question the legal authority for requiring such access. The general constitutional underpinnings discussed above provide the foundation for federal and state statutes and regulations that govern the conduct of health officials directing an epidemiologic investigation. For epidemiologists employed by the federal government, the laws relating to the general powers and duties of the PHS for research and investigation are found in Title III of the Public Health Service Act. The general statutory authority that is applicable to federal epidemiologic investigations is Section 301 of the Public Health Service Act, 42 U.S.C. 241:

> The Secretary shall conduct in the Service, and encourage, cooperate with, and render assistance to other appropriate public authorities, scientific institutions, and scientists in the conduct of, and promote the coordination of, research, investigations, experiments, demonstrations, and studies relating to the causes, diagnosis, treatment, control, and prevention of physical and mental diseases and impairments of man. . . . [42 U.S.C. 241(a), (emphasis added).]

In addition, subsection 6 of Section 301 indicates that the secretary is authorized to "make available, to health officials, scientists, and appropriate public and other nonprofit institutions and organizations, technical advice and assistance on the application of statistical methods to experiments, studies, and surveys in health and medical fields." Although these provisions of Section 301 are broadly worded and are permissive rather than compulsory, they nonetheless give legal authority for intervention by federal epidemiologists in disease outbreaks and other instances in which such assistance is requested.

As mentioned previously, individual states and local jurisdictions will have various laws and regulations that authorize or relate to the conduct of public health investigations. However, state laws regarding compelling access to facilities and records are generally more specific and likely have provisions that compel cooperation within the boundaries of due process.

COLLECTING DATA

The process of collecting data during an epidemiologic field investigation involves a number of legal considerations, including the following: (1) protection available under state or federal law during and after the investigation for the records collected and generated in relation to the investigation; (2) special confidentiality provisions for medical or other information; (3) required reporting of particular diseases or conditions; (4) status of information in investigative files under the federal Freedom of Information Act (FOIA) (5 U.S.C. Section 552) or state FOIA counterparts; and (5) the applicability of federal or state human subjects research regulations, including the need for review of study protocols by institutional review boards and the need for informed consent for participation in the investigation or for procedures related to the investigation.

Protection of Investigational Records

To determine what records will be kept or generated and where and how such records will be stored, you need to know what legal protection is in place for the documents and other records that will be examined, extracted, and compiled in association with the investigation. Most states provide specific statutory and regulatory confidentiality protection over medical and public health records. In general, the confidentiality protection prevents the disclosure of a name-identified record without the consent of the person on whom the record is maintained. Accordingly, such medical records in the hands of an investigator are generally protected by state law. Furthermore, such state laws frequently require that only certain authorized personnel have access to such confidential records and that such records be maintained in a secure manner. You would usually be authorized to have access to such records but would be bound to maintain the records in a manner that would protect the confidentiality of the identifiable information from unauthorized or inadvertent disclosure.

In the course of an investigation, you may create or compile a number of documents (e.g., questionnaires, forms, investigative notes, copies or extractions of patient or other records, letters, reports, memoranda, drafts, manuscripts, and final reports). Depending on the nature of the records and the status of the investigation, these documents may not be protected from disclosure to the public by state or federal laws. Except for records afforded specific protection by state or federal laws (such as state laws protecting medical records), you should probably assume that all records collected may at some point be open to public scrutiny.

Investigators who are federal employees need to be aware of the provisions of the Freedom of Information Act (FOIA), 5 U.S.C. Section 552. In general, the FOIA provides that all documents in the hands of federal employees, on federal premises, or within the control of federal employees are available to the public unless specifically exempted by the act. The act contains nine exemptions. In general, four of these exemptions may affect epidemiologic investigations.

Interagency and intraagency communications

Exemption (b)(5) permits the federal government to withhold from disclosure interagency and intraagency memorandums or letters that would not be available "to a party other than an agency in litigation with the agency." An example of the use of this exemption would be to protect from disclosure a draft memorandum written by the investigator to his or her supervisor describing the early findings of the investigation.

Personnel and medical records

Exemption (b)(6) permits the federal government to withhold from mandatory disclosure "personnel and medical files and similar files the disclosure of which would constitute a clearly unwarranted invasion of personal privacy." This exemption may be invoked by the federal government to protect confidential medical information on an individual contained in a record collected by the federal investigator.

Information otherwise exempt from disclosure by statute

Exemption (b)(3) provides that a federal agency may withhold from disclosure information "specifically exempted from disclosure by statute." If an epidemiologic investigation is conducted under an assurance of confidentiality authorized by a federal statute (such as Section 301(d) or Section 308(d) of the Public Health Service Act), the information collected pursuant to the confidentiality assurance is protected from disclosure under the FOIA in a manner that would contravene the statutory provision. Sections 301(d) and 308(d) are similar to provisions for certificates of confidentiality for federally funded alcohol and drug abuse patient records under 42 C.F.R. Part 2. You should be aware that such assurances of confidentiality are not commonly used. Instead, with legal counsel and on a case-by-case basis, such assurances are limited to exceptional circumstances in which the sensitivity of the information demands additional confidentiality measures or when the cooperation of the study subjects would be impeded in the absence of such an assurance.

Trade secrets and commercial or financial information

Exemption (b)(4) permits the federal government " to withhold from disclosure commercial or financial information obtained from a person and privileged and confidential." Although this exemption may be less commonly applicable than the other three outlined above, it would be relevant to an epidemiologic investigation which involved, for example, a commercial product on which the investigator has records containing trade secrets or confidential information on the components of the product. Likewise, confidential financial information may be contained in investigative records, even records that might otherwise be disclosed under the FOIA.

Disease Reporting

Within the realm of collecting information, you must be aware of the public health responsibilities regarding disease reporting to appropriate authorities. While the diagnosis of reportable diseases more commonly occurs in the treatment setting, it is possible that your investigation may identify a reportable disease or a previously diagnosed condition that has not been reported. Accordingly, you should be knowledgeable about disease reporting requirements in the jurisdiction in which the investigation is being conducted and should be prepared either to make such reports, if appropriate, or to see that the report is made by the responsible person or institution.

Research Involving Human Subjects

Federal employees and those supported by federal funds for the investigation should be aware of the provisions of the federal regulations governing the Protection of Human Subjects, 45 C.F.R. Part 46. Although you may question whether your investigation constitutes "research," the definition for research under Part 46 is specific: "'Research' means a systematic investigation designed to develop or contribute to generalizable knowledge." This definition is very inclusive of activities that may include surveillance, outbreak investigations, and other public health interventions. However, Part 46 also provides certain exceptions for "research involving survey or interview procedures," including an exception if the responses are recorded without identifiers. Accordingly, when you plan your field investigation, be aware of the provisions of 45 C.F.R. Part 46.

The requirements regarding informed consent of individuals who are interviewed or studied in a field investigation are usually a matter of state law in the jurisdiction in which the investigation takes place. However, 45 C.F.R. 46.116 outlines the circumstances that require written or oral informed consent if Health and Human Services Administration funds support the research activity. The Part 46 regulations also describe the basic elements of informed consent, including information on benefits and risks of participation that must be disclosed to research subjects.

Privacy Act

The federal Privacy Act, 5 U.S.C. 552a, is applicable to any investigation conducted by a federal employee and to the retention of personally identifiable records retained within a federal "system of records." The Privacy Act generally allows an individual to have access to his or her records held by a federal agency. Certain national security and criminal law enforcement records are exempt from the Privacy Act.

In addition, federal agencies must publish notices describing all systems of records and must make reasonable efforts to maintain accurate, relevant, and timely information. Information collected for one purpose must not be used for another purpose without notice to or the consent of the individual on whom the record is maintained.

The Privacy Act applies only to records containing personal identifiers. Accordingly, you should consider whether there is a valid need to retain identifying information. For example, the CDC pledges that records containing names and other identifiers will be retained only when necessary, and only with identifiers as long as necessary. Violations of the Privacy Act are punishable by civil and criminal penalties.

THE EPIDEMIOLOGIST AND LITIGATION

Occasionally, you may conduct an investigation that results in the need for intervention by federal or state law enforcement authorities. In this circumstance, you must be aware of other legal considerations. For example, epidemiologic investigations of clusters of deaths of hospitalized patients have led to homicide and assault prosecution of nurses who had cared for the deceased patients. Studies of deaths in a pediatric intensive-care unit led to action by the Food and Drug

Administration against the manufacturer and distributor of an infant feeding formula.

The realm of enforcement actions will place you in somewhat unfamiliar territory. For the epidemiologist trained to collect and analyze data objectively and quantitatively, the partiality of the advocacy role of attorneys can be frustrating. Although epidemiologists are more comfortable with probabilities, associations, and confidence intervals for populations, attorneys usually seek cause and effect for an individual. While the epidemiologist seeks to retain the appropriate terminology for the conclusions, prosecutors may hope to portray the findings as definitive rather than circumstantial. The enforcement arena likewise places the epidemiologist in a potential new role—that of a witness. The scrutiny you are subjected to in the peer review process may be comfortably familiar, but the scrutiny of the same scientific data in an enforcement proceeding is less predictable.

Attorneys are advocates who take an oath to pursue the case of their client vigorously. Understandably, then, situations involving formal encounters with attorneys for either side in a controversy are seldom impartial or dispassionate. Whether in administrative hearings, depositions, or court proceedings, witnesses are questioned by one side and then cross-examined by the attorney for the other side. The purpose of cross-examination is generally to minimize, discredit, or at least limit the effect of the testimony given on direct examination. The prospect that a nonscientist will scrutinize the data in a manner that appears more to be twisting, stretching, and perhaps even misconstruing is usually disconcerting to the epidemiologist as a witness. If you believe you can provide an impartial, independent third-party view to a legal forum, you may find yourself ensnared by adversaries, legal objections, judges, and rules of procedure. However, the unfamiliarity of the forum does not obviate your responsibility to assure the public's health.

INTERVENTION

Compulsory Measures

The state's ability to carry out its role in protecting the public health strongly depends on the cooperation of citizens in voluntarily complying with the various disease control standards and good public health practices. Nonetheless, the state's broad police powers also include the power to compel persons in certain circumstances to undergo medical examinations, vaccinations, and testing and to require quarantine or isolation of persons who may pose a threat to the public because they have a particular communicable disease. Most states have general public health laws and regulations that enumerate the compulsory powers and the procedures associated with the exercise of those compulsory powers. In addition to the general compulsory public health statutes and regulations on compulsory powers and duties, however, most states also have laws that are specific to the control of tuberculosis and sexually transmissible diseases.

The following are examples of compulsory procedures that have been upheld by the courts: requirements for immunization prior to school attendance; preemployment screening for communicable diseases such as tuberculosis or in occupations where the individual will have contact with the public; compulsory treatment of persons with active tuberculosis; mandatory examinations or screening of marriage license applicants; laws or ordinances mandating compliance with sanitation standards in public and private buildings; closing of bathhouses to prevent high-risk sexual activity; and the authority to institutionalize, involuntarily, individuals in certain situations (most often mental illness or drug abuse).

Isolation and Quarantine

As indicated previously, state laws have provisions for stricter methods of disease control than are generally used in current public health practice. Federal law and laws in all states still provide authority for quarantine for certain communicable diseases. In addition, some states have enacted laws that provide specific authority for quarantine and isolation of persons with human immunodeficiency virus (HIV) or acquired immunodeficiency syndrome (AIDS). Quarantine usually involves complete restriction of the patient and the household contacts of the patient to the location where the patient is receiving care. These laws, written decades ago, usually still contain enumeration of such requirements as posting of a placard to warn other persons against entering the quarantined area.

Federal and state courts have upheld quarantine statutes as a valid exercise of the state's police power. The U.S. Supreme Court in the case of *Jacobson* v. *Massachusetts* (discussed previously) held that states have the authority to enact quarantine and other health laws as means of protecting the community against communicable diseases. Likewise, other state and federal courts have followed the rationale of the Jacobson case and have uniformly upheld state quarantine statutes in the context of communicable disease control.

Quarantine of persons with venereal disease and HIV have also been upheld. The U.S. Court of Appeals for the Tenth Circuit in *Reynolds* v. *McNichols*, 488 F.2d 1378 (10th Cir. 1973), ruled that quarantining and compelling treatment of persons with venereal disease was a proper exercise of the state's police power. State courts in Florida, California, and Nevada have used quarantine statutes to detain HIV-infected prostitutes. In one case in Florida that received significant press coverage, an AIDS-infected female prostitute was ordered to stay in her home and was forced to wear an electronic device that would signal police if she traveled more than 200 feet from her telephone. In 1983, a New York State court held that the state could quarantine prisoners who had AIDS because the actions by corrections authorities constituted a reasonable measure to stop HIV transmission in the prison population [*LaRocca v. Dalsheim*, 120 Misc.2d 697, 467 N.Y.S. 2d 302 (N.Y. Sup. 1983)].

The exercise of the state's public health powers, including quarantine and isolation, is limited by constraints that are part of the federal and state constitutions. These provisions place both procedural and substantive safeguards that limit the state's exercise of police power. The courts have mandated that the state exercise its police power using the "least restrictive alternative" when depriving an individual of liberty while pursuing a valid state interest. The use of the least restrictive alternative represents a balancing of the public health interests with the individual's deprivation of personal liberty. Most notably, the use of the least restrictive alternative has developed in situations involving civil commitment proceedings. Similarly, application of this principle to quarantine law enforcement may provide for compliance with a regimen of care under the supervision of a physician rather than mandatory hospitalization.

SUMMARY

As has been discussed, the field epidemiologist should understand that the basic authority of public health officials to conduct investigations of disease or epidemic outbreaks is the state's inherent police powers. Federal and state laws governing the health and safety of the public are enacted pursuant to this broad authority. These laws provide not only for the state to have access to medical and other records for purposes of public health investigations but also for protection of the individual's interest in privacy by placing strict limits on access to medical, hospital, and public health records. While public health investigations and activities usually rely on the voluntary cooperation of individuals and institutions, federal and state laws provide authority for the use of compulsory measures, when necessary, for the protection of the public health and safety.

Field epidemiologists are not expected to know public health law. Yet they should have an appreciation of the legal issues that pertain to surveillance, confidentiality of medical records, and the legal responsibilities of both federal and state governments. The quality, quantity, and ease of collecting epidemiologic data can be enhanced materially by an awareness of these issues and, if necessary, consultation with the legal profession.

FURTHER READING

Gostin, L. (1989). The politics of AIDS: Compulsory state powers, public health and civil liberties. *49 Ohio State Law Journal 1017*.

Grad, F. P. (1990). *The public health law manual* (2nd ed.). The American Public Health Association, Washington, D.C.

Wing, K. R. (1990). *The law and the public's health* (3rd ed.). Health Administration Press, Ann Arbor, Michigan.

15

INVESTIGATIONS IN
HEALTH CARE FACILITIES

Stephanie Zaza
William R. Jarvis

The purpose of this chapter is to prepare you for field investigations in health care facilities. The chapter highlights the differences between conducting a community outbreak investigation and an outbreak investigation confined to a health care facility; the emphasis is on how to find the information you need and how to use data and resources that are readily available in health care settings.

The term "health care facility" refers to hospitals, private physicians' offices, freestanding clinics, and long-term-care facilities (Table 15–1). Investigations of outbreaks in health care facilities require special attention and differ from those of community outbreaks in several ways.

BACKGROUND CONSIDERATIONS

Community- versus Hospital-Based Outbreaks

Nosocomial infections (e.g., hospital-acquired bloodstream, respiratory, urinary tract, and surgical wound infections) are common, occurring in approximately 6 percent of hospitalized patients.[1] Of every 1,000 hospitalized patients, urinary tract infections occur in an estimated 24, nosocomial pneumonia in 6 to 10, and bloodstream infections in 3. Further, surgical wound infections result from 28 of

Table 15–1. Health Care Facilities

Hospitals

Private physicians' offices

Freestanding clinics
  Dialysis
  Ambulatory surgery

Long-term-care facilities
  Nursing homes
  Rehabilitation centers
  Institutions for the mentally or physically handicapped

---

every 1,000 operations performed.[1,2] Although it is possible that approximately 32 percent of nosocomial infections could be prevented by using current recommendations, only 6 percent actually *are* prevented.[3] Most nosocomial infections are endemic; epidemics of hospital infection are infrequent.[4] Outbreaks of infections in health care facilities, when they do occur, involve a wide range of infectious agents and sites: Outbreaks of noninfectious diseases also occur in health care facilities. There have been recent investigations of outbreaks of such infectious and noninfectious problems as gram-negative bacteremia in dialysis or intensive care unit patients, aspergillosis among immunosuppressed patients, surgical wound infections after breast implants, tuberculosis among patients and health care workers (HCWs), anaphylactic reactions to latex among pediatric surgery patients, and aluminum toxicity among dialysis patients[5–11,18] (also CDC, unpublished data).

Hospitalized patients, residents of long-term-care facilities, and chronic hemodialysis patients have underlying diseases that make them highly susceptible to infection. Other risk factors for the development of infection may include invasive procedures, intravenous catheters, indwelling urinary catheters, and endotracheal intubation. These numerous, interacting risk factors add complexity to the investigation and may require multivariate analyses to reduce or eliminate the effect of confounding variables and to identify the independent risk factor or factors.

Hospital pathogens such as multidrug-resistant *Mycobacterium tuberculosis*, methicillin-resistant *Staphylococcus aureus*, hepatitis B virus, and other microorganisms also pose a risk to HCWs in these facilities. Nosocomial transmission is often evidenced by infections among both HCWs and patients.

Finally, any outbreak of nosocomially transmitted disease poses the risk of litigation against the health care facility. This increases the pressure to identify the problem rapidly and to institute effective control measures during the investigation.

Overall Purposes

As with community outbreak investigations, the primary purpose of epidemiologic investigations in health care facilities is to determine the source of the outbreak and prevent further spread of disease. Investigations provide the opportunity to identify new or reemerging agents or complications, previously unrecognized human or environmental sources, and new or unusual modes of transmission. Likewise, investigations in health care facilities may help determine risk factors for the development of disease in patients and/or HCWs.

Pace and Commitment of the Field Investigation

Like most epidemiologic investigation in the field, studies in health care facilities must be conducted quickly and responsibly. Pressure from a variety of sources may add to the sense of urgency to complete the investigation quickly. First, health care professionals will be looking to you for answers and recommendations to prevent further spread of disease to their "healthy" patients and/or to HCWs. Second, the hospital administrators may already have stopped admissions to the affected unit; every day that unit stays closed means loss of income for the hospital. Finally, the health care industry is a common target of the media; outbreaks in a health care facility may lead to adverse publicity for the facility. Yet these added pressures should not affect the conduct or organization of your investigation. Although you can make preliminary recommendations based on sound infection control practices, such as patient isolation and/or hand washing, collect your data carefully, analyze it appropriately, and then make specific recommendations based on your findings. Subsequent decisions to reverse actions taken by the health care facility before your arrival (e.g., closing a certain ward to all admissions) should be made by the personnel of the health care facility.

RECOGNITION AND RESPONSE TO A REQUEST FOR ASSISTANCE

The Report

The Joint Commission on Accreditation of Healthcare Organizations (JCAHO) requires that health care facilities maintain an active infection control program, including surveillance for nosocomial infections, as a part of their standard for being accredited.[12] Surveillance data serve as a source for the identification of infectious disease outbreaks and as a measurement of the intensity and efficacy of the facility's infection surveillance and control program. With caution, these data can also be used to monitor infection rates by comparing the facility's rates over time with those of similar facilities.

Practitioners trained in infection control techniques monitor infections in hospitalized patients. These infection control practitioners (ICPs) also may work in freestanding clinics and/or long-term-care facilities. They conduct routine surveillance for nosocomial infections, usually using uniform definitions.[13] Common sources for surveillance data are the microbiology laboratory; medical, pharmacy, radiology, and Kardex-medical records; nursing, surgical service, and physician reports; and discharge summaries. Reports of outbreaks in health care facilities often result from analysis of these surveillance data. Reports of a possible outbreak may come from an ICP who calls the local or state health department or CDC asking for advice on infection control practices. Possible outbreaks may also be recognized by microbiology laboratories, physicians, employee health departments or by employees, patients, patients' families, or the news media.

The health care facility or the local health department may indicate the existence of an outbreak by asking for laboratory support from the state health department or the CDC. When a request for laboratory support is received, one may identify an outbreak by asking for more information. This, in turn, might generate a request for assistance.

The Request

Requests for epidemiologic assistance usually come from the ICP, the hospital epidemiologist, the facility's administrator, or a private physician who has an outbreak in her or his office. The personnel of the health care facility may simply need laboratory support, may lack epidemiologic expertise, or may be too understaffed to conduct an investigation on their own while still performing their usual duties. Inquiries about possible assistance may be guarded because of concern over potential future litigation or adverse publicity.

The Response and the Responsibilities

A request to investigate an outbreak in a health care facility does not guarantee that an investigation will be performed. Because infections and other complications are so common in health care facilities, you should get additional background information before agreeing to initiate an investigation. For example, if you receive a call requesting assistance in determining the source of surgical wound infections among open-heart surgery (OHS) patients during the previous 2 months, try to get additional information that may be useful in evaluating the need for assistance. This information could include current and background OHS wound-infection rates, the pathogens causing infection and whether isolates are available, and a line listing of cases and their characteristics and risk factors. Always ask if the "outbreak" isolates are available; this is particularly important for confirming the identity of infecting strains and for laboratory typing, which are often essential for conclusive epidemiologic investigations of a nosocomial outbreak.

Second, ask the contact person to determine the OHS wound-infection rate among patients for several months to years before the possible outbreak. From this rate, determine if an outbreak may, indeed, be occurring or if the health care facility actually has a high endemic rate. Determine if the increased OHS wound-infection rate could be due to surveillance artifact. For example, has there been an increase in the surveillance staff or training of new infection control personnel? Have there been additions to the OHS staff or changes in practices such as the introduction of a new technique or changes in the types of procedures performed or patients treated? Are there any changes in the laboratory that would bring about increased recognition of the pathogens? If an increase in the rate of OHS wound infections can be temporally linked to an increase in one of these factors, a full on-site investigation may not be necessary. Finally, ask about any interim infection control measures that may have been put into place. If good infection control practices have been implemented and the problem persists, an investigation may be warranted.

Before beginning an investigation, participants need to discuss several critical issues. These issues include organization, personnel, resources, and responsibilities (see Chapter 4).

PREPARATION FOR THE FIELD INVESTIGATION

Collaboration and Consultation

Investigations of infectious disease outbreaks in health care settings usually require substantial laboratory support. In addition to identifying the agent (which may already have been done by the health care facility), further typing of the organism may be necessary. For example, since many serotypes of *Pseudomonas aeruginosa* exist as common environmental organisms in hospitals, outbreaks of *P. aeruginosa* may require serotyping to link patient and environmental isolates. Also, serologic testing of numerous specimens may be required in outbreaks of nosocomially transmitted viral infections, such as hepatitis A, B, or C and cytomegalovirus. Typing methods vary from organism to organism (Table 15–2). Excepting antimicrobial susceptibility testing, most typing methods are available only in reference laboratories. Before leaving for the field, your reference laboratory should be contacted to notify them that an outbreak investigation will be starting; to identify a contact person in the laboratory, and to determine what types of specimens should be collected, how they should be shipped, and what capabilities the laboratory has for this particular investigation. The labora-

Table 15–2. Types of Organisms for Which Typing Method Can Be Used

TYPING METHODS	TYPES OF ORGANISMS
Antimicrobial susceptibility profiles	Bacteria (except *Pseudomonas cepacia* and *Staphylococcus epidermidis*), fungi, occasionally viruses
Serotyping	Some bacteria and viruses
Pulsed-field gel electrophoresis	Bacteria and fungi
Ribotyping	Bacteria
Phage typing	Bacteria (i.e., *Staphylococcus aureus*)
Plasmid analysis	Bacteria
Restriction fragment length polymorphism	*Mycobacterium tuberculosis*

tory should also be able to estimate a time frame for results. A more comprehensive discussion of the laboratory's role in investigating outbreaks can be found in Chapter 18.

For outbreaks involving medical products, devices, biologicals, or blood products, the Food and Drug Administration (FDA) should be notified and consulted for laws requiring the reporting of adverse effects. In addition, the FDA may have been notified of a similar problem from other facilities, indicating a problem of potentially greater scope. The FDA can issue alerts and product recalls to the medical community if such a problem occurs. Similarly, for outbreaks primarily involving HCWs or physical plant problems (e.g., potential toxic exposure among HCWs), state agencies responsible for occupational health and/or the National Institute for Occupational Safety and Health (NIOSH) can lend assistance with industrial engineering evaluations.

In contrast to community outbreak investigators, the epidemiologist often has assistance from ICPs knowledgeable about the health care facility and trained in hospital infection control practices. These ICPs are an invaluable resource for background information about infection rates at the facility and for assistance with the location of other resources that may be available to you. In addition, the ICP's staff may be available to assist with abstraction of medical records after you have determined what information will be collected.

Health care facilities want to minimize the potentially negative impact that an investigation may generate. Public inquiries will be inevitable and should be handled by the administrative, public relations, or risk-management personnel at the facility. In addition to allowing you to conduct the investigation unhindered by the media, this allows the facility to maintain control of this very delicate aspect of the investigation.

THE FIELD INVESTIGATION

Health care facilities lend themselves to outbreak investigations because they provide easy access to many kinds of records (see above). Documentation is very important in health care facilities, but it varies; hospitals and freestanding clinics (surgery or dialysis centers) generally have more complete documentation than do long-term-care facilities and private physicians' offices. Use your imagination to identify other sources of documentation and do not be afraid to ask if other types of records exist. Outbreaks predominantly involving HCWs are more difficult because not all of the HCWs will be treated at the health care facility. Employee health department records can be used, although medical students, house officers, outside agency personnel, volunteers, and other unpaid hospital personnel are often not included in hospital employee health programs. Time cards (to determine absenteeism possibly due to illness) and interviews with affected employees are also helpful.

Immediately upon your arrival at the health care facility, arrange a meeting with all of the key personnel involved with the outbreak. This meeting should include the hospital administrator, chief of service, and/or any physicians who have patients involved in the outbreak, the hospital epidemiologist and the infection control staff, risk-management personnel, appropriate public health authorities, and the field team. Also invite any other key personnel who may be involved, such as the operating room manager, the head nurse from the affected unit, and the head of the microbiology department. At this meeting, you should outline your initial plan for the investigation and request any resources you need immediately: an office with a telephone, phone numbers of key personnel, a map of the facility, and directions to the laboratory and medical records department. If security is strict in the facility, request a temporary identification badge to allow freer access to the facility. Also, ask for any additional information you may need to start the investigation—for example, policy and procedure changes and impressions as to the possible cause of the outbreak. Introductions to the chiefs of the affected services will garner cooperation from their staffs. It is also important to confirm that you will maintain the strictest confidentiality for the patients and will work with the health care facility personnel to conduct the investigation quickly and efficiently, with as little disruption of usual business as possible.

Determine the Existence of an Epidemic

This step may have been started during the preparatory stages of the investigation (see Chapter 5). In the field, determine the background rate of infections for yourself. Start with microbiology and infection control records if applicable. Outbreaks involving blood products will require examination of transfusion reaction records;

those involving dialysis patients require examination of dialysis session records. Be creative—what you need is not always computerized but is often systematically logged somewhere. You may have to look back at several years of data to calculate accurate background rates. If the data suggest a hyperendemic rate rather than a true outbreak, the problem still may be worthy of investigation. Remember to look at other changes that may have occurred that will affect the rates you are calculating (e.g., the ICP hired six new assistants one year, or four new surgeons or a new infectious disease specialist were added to the medical staff). New procedures may have been implemented before or during the outbreak, new diagnostic tests may have become available, or new units may have been opened in the hospital—all of which might lead to an increased infection rate.

At the same time, start looking closely at procedures around the patient-care areas that are relevant to the outbreak. Look at everything and ask questions about every aspect of patient care no matter how seemingly trivial. See for yourself what is actually happening rather than relying on others. Policies that are written on paper may or may not reflect what is really occurring on the patient-care wards. After your initial review of the procedures occurring around the patients, create your initial case definition and determine what data you want to collect for each case. For example, patient demographic information, hospital location, underlying diagnoses, date of onset of illness, and dates of invasive procedures should be collected. Other important data might include severity-of-illness indicators [e.g., the Acute Physiologic and Chronic Health Evaluation (APACHE) score, the Pediatric Risk of Mortality (PRISM) score, or the National Nosocomial Infections Surveillance surgical wound infection risk index],[14-16] operating room, surgeon, operating room team members, nursing and other patient contact personnel, and medications.

Confirm the Diagnosis

In an infectious disease outbreak, confirm that the cases are related by using the hospital microbiology laboratory to perform species identification and/or antimicrobial sensitivity testing if possible. For typing of organisms beyond the capability of the microbiology department at the facility, consult the local or state health department laboratory. Remember, some typing techniques are research tools that cannot be performed rapidly and/or may not be practical to apply to large numbers of isolates. Call your laboratory contact as early as possible to request assistance and discuss a reasonable time frame for results.

Define a Case and Count Cases

The case definitions should start with the clinical aspects of the disease. Try to include clinical and laboratory data in the case definition as well as inclusionary characteristics that relate to time, place, and person. For example, a case definition might include persons who developed a staphylococcal wound infection between November 1 and January 1; who were located on surgical floor 3-West; and who had an orthopedic procedure. If the diagnosis is easily and quickly confirmed by laboratory methods, the confirmation criteria can be used to define a *confirmed* case; patients with symptoms but lacking laboratory confirmation can be referred to as *possible* cases. Remember, start with a broad case definition; you can refine it as you continue the investigation.

Methods for case finding depend on the type of disease (infectious or noninfectious) causing the outbreak. Sources that may be useful include microbiology, infection control surveillance, transfusion, emergency room, clinic patient, or dialysis session records. Case finding by reviewing the entire cohort of patient charts can be done if the cases are limited to a single ward or unit or if the health care facility is very small (i.e., with a total number of charts that can be reviewed in a reasonable period of time). Dialysis outbreaks may require that each patient not be counted as a single case; rather, each dialysis session for a patient may have to be counted if an exposure may have occurred during one or more of many sessions. This allows each dialysis session to be treated as a single exposure.

At the same time you are ascertaining cases, collect the basic information you have already deemed important during your initial procedure review of the originally identified cases. Again, after you have determined your case definition and found cases, compare the attack rate with the background rate to assure yourself that an outbreak is indeed occurring.

Orient the Data in Terms of Time, Place, and Person

Descriptive epidemiology in health care facilities differs from that in community outbreak investigations only in that all of the cases have been hospitalized or have visited a clinic or a physician's office. As with community outbreaks, organizing the data in terms of time, place, and person allows you to postulate who was at risk, who may still be at risk, and what the critical exposure was.

Time

The "epidemic curve" gives you a picture of the scope of the outbreak over time. It may offer a clue as to whether the outbreak was due to a common source, person-to-person transmission, or another mode of transmission (see Chapter 6). For example, a common-source outbreak with subsequent person-to-person transmission is well illustrated by a food-borne outbreak in a retirement community (Figure 15–1). A high initial peak of onset of illness, suggestive of a single point source of infection, is followed by continued cases of illness due to secondary person-to-person transmission typical of outbreaks of viral gastroenteritis. The epidemic curve

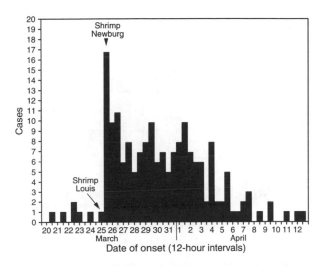

Figure 15-1. Cases of gastroenteritis originating from a common source with subsequent person-to-person transmission, by date of onset—California, March 20–April 12, 1988. *Source*: Gordon et al. (1990).[17]

of an outbreak caused by contaminated patient equipment or poor infection control techniques may also span long periods of time until the recurring problem is corrected. For example, an *Acinetobacter baumannii* outbreak related to reusable intravascular transducers that were not adequately sterilized continued for over a year until the problem was recognized and the decontamination/disinfection technique corrected (Figure 15-2).[18] If HCWs and patients are both affected by the outbreak, the date of onset of disease for patients and HCWs should be plotted together and separately to help determine how transmission may have occurred: from patient to patient, patient to HCW, HCW to patient, or HCW to HCW.

Place

At times, the location of the outbreak will be limited to a certain floor, unit, or operating room; at other times a certain type of activity will be involved (e.g., all of the general surgical units because only surgical patients are being affected). The location of the outbreak may provide a clue to the mode of transmission or to certain risk factors stemming from patient placement. For example, in a hospital with high rates of tuberculin skin test conversion among its patients and HCWs, an investigation revealed that many of the skin test converters were exposed to AIDS patients with active tuberculosis in the outpatient HIV clinic.[19] In that investigation, the location of cases identified risk factors for acquisition of the disease—exposure in a clinic to patients with active tuberculosis, and to mode of transmission—airborne spread due to poor isolation techniques.

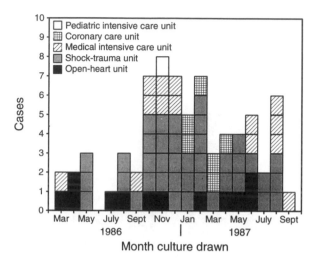

Figure 15-2. Cases of *Acinetobacter baumannii* bacteria caused by contaminated patient care equiptment, by month culture was drawn and hospital ward—New Jersey, March 1986–September 1987. *Source:* Beck-Sague et al. (1990).[18]

Person

In investigating communitywide epidemics, you will often characterize the affected persons by many attributes such as age, gender, race, occupation, socio-economic level, religion, immune status, and the like. In general, however, in health care settings, you do not need to classify cases by so many variables. Generally, age, gender, and underlying disease are the most often used attributes that help you define the "at-risk" population.

Determine Who Is at Risk of Becoming Ill

As discussed in previous chapters (see Chapter 6), the purpose of characterizing the ill persons by time, place, and person is to give you an idea of who is at risk of disease and whom to study further. Therefore, either examine the entire population for a retrospective cohort study or randomly select controls from this population for a case-control study (see Chapter 7). If, for example, you find that patients located on all general wards of the hospital over a period of 1 year developed pneumonia, you may want to take a random sample of all patients admitted to the hospital during that same year as controls for a case-control study. If, however, you determine that the only patients in the facility who are at risk were located on a particular ward during a specific time interval and had a particular underlying diagnosis (e.g., appendectomy patients on a general surgical ward during the months of April and May 1992), you may want to select all appendectomy patients located on that ward from March 1 through June 30, 1992, and review their charts as a retrospective cohort study.

Selection of controls is exceedingly important, because the wrong control group can easily lead to erroneous conclusions. For example, if, during case finding, you discover that patients undergoing general anesthesia for a variety of surgical procedures developed surgical wound and bloodstream infections, several possible control groups for a case-control study could be selected, as well as several different cohorts. If the study group (controls or the cohort) is selected from all patients undergoing surgery, there is a good chance that many of the non-ill patients will have undergone local, spinal, or epidural anesthesia, while all of the ill patients will have undergone only general anesthesia. Since the ill patients were previously known to have undergone only general anesthesia, specific exposures related to general anesthesia (e.g., particular injectable anesthetics or intubation equipment) probably will not be identified with this group of controls. A better study group would include patients undergoing general anesthesia for surgical procedures during the correct time frame. This will allow analysis of each individual injectable and inhalational agent, respiratory equipment, anesthesiologist, and other possible risk factors.

Develop and Test Hypotheses

It is often inefficient to test only one or two hypotheses at a time. Test several factors at once by collecting data on cases and controls or the cohort that examine several risks. For example, if the disease is predominantly spread by the respiratory route and all of the cases were intubated, you may want to examine all respiratory therapy practices and exposures, including the type of ventilator used, duration of ventilation, which respiratory therapist took care of the cases each shift, which nurses suctioned the patients' endotracheal tubes, which medications were administered through the endotracheal tube and who prepared them, and how often the ventilator reservoirs were changed.

An excellent example of an outbreak investigation in a hospital is the investigation of surgical wound infections caused by an unusual human pathogen, *Rhodococcus bronchialis*, after open-heart surgery.[20] This outbreak provided an opportunity to assess risk factors for infection with *R. bronchialis*, mode of transmission of the organism, and potential sources of this unusual nosocomial-pathogen. Logical hypotheses for the source of surgical wound infections after open-heart surgery included the preoperative (e.g., nurses, physicians, wards), operative (e.g., operating room environment or personnel), and postoperative (e.g., recovery room or intensive care unit personnel) exposures. By retrospective cohort analysis, the investigators analyzed a large number of variables as measures of potential risk for infection and possible exposures as the source of infection

(Table 15–3). The only factor significantly associated with infection was the presence of one operating room nurse, nurse A, during the operative procedure. Examination of nurse A's intraoperative practices revealed that she could potentially contaminate the sterile field after performing an activated clotting-time test that involved the use of a water bath for incubation of a tube of the patient's blood. The hypothesis was that nurse A contaminated the sterile operative field after performing the test; this would account for all of the cases of *R. bronchialis* surgical wound infections during the epidemic period.

Compare the Hypothesis with the Established Facts

Environmental and personnel cultures can help support the results of an epidemiologic investigation. Because many organisms are ubiquitous in health care environments and are part of the normal human flora, performing cultures of the environment or personnel without epidemiologic implications can waste precious time and lead your investigation astray. However, when performed to determine whether your epidemiologic data are pointing you in the right direction, environmental and personnel cultures can be very valuable.

To continue with the previous example, in order to establish that nurse A was, indeed, responsible for all of the cases of *R. bronchialis* at the hospital, the investigators performed numerous cultures as indicated by the epidemiologic data. These included cultures of nurse A and nurse B's hands before and after each performed the activated clotting-time test; nasal swabs from all cardiac operating room personnel; swabs from nurse A's scalp, pharynx, vagina, and rectum; swabs of the neck-scruff skin, mouths, rectums, and paws of two of nurse A's three dogs; and environmental swabs while nurse A was present in and absent from the operating room. Only cultures of nurse A's hands after performing the activated clotting test, nurse A's nasal swab, settle plates from the operating room while nurse A was present, nurse A's scalp and vaginal cultures, and material from the neck-scruff skin of nurse A's dogs were positive for *R. bronchialis*. Antimicrobial sensitivity testing, plasmid analysis, and restriction fragment length polymorphism analysis showed that all of the outbreak isolates were identical and distinct from nonoutbreak stock isolates.

The role of the water bath used to incubate blood samples for the activated clotting-time test was analyzed by using a colorless fluorescent dye. After simulating the beginning of an open-heart procedure, 8 of 11 circulating nurses had "contaminated" the sterile field with fluorescent dye from the water bath. In addition, all of the nurses' hands; some of the nurses' wrists, forearms, and scrub suits; the outer surface of the water bath container; the table surface; and the floor around the water bath were "contaminated" with fluorescent dye. This experiment showed that although the bath water was culture-negative for *R. bronchialis*, the water

Table 15–3. Potential Risk Factors for Rhodococcus Sternal Wound Infection—
May 1 through December 31, 1988[a]

POTENTIAL RISK FACTOR	CASE PATIENTS $(N = 7)$	CONTROLS $(N = 28)$	ODDS RATIO	P VALUES
Categorical Variables				
Male sex	7 (100)	24 (86)	NC	0.6
Underlying conditions	6 (86)	22 (79)	1.6	1.0
Diabetes	1 (14)	6 (21)	0.6	0.1
Obesity	3 (43)	4 (14)	4.5	0.1
Smoking	4 (57)	9 (32)	2.8	0.4
Cancer	1 (14)	0 (0)	NC	0.2
Renal insufficiency	0 (0)	0 (0)	—	—
Treatment with steroids	1 (14)	1 (4)	4.5	0.4
Chronic lung disease	2 (29)	3 (11)	3.3	0.3
Presence of nurse A	7 (100)	6 (21)	NC	0.0003
Coronary artery bypass graft	7 (100)	28 (100)	—	—
Saphenous vein	6 (86)	26 (93)	0.5	0.5
Mammary artery	6 (86)	25 (89)	0.7	1.0
Transfusion	4 (57)	13 (46)	2.2	1.0
Continuous Variables				
Preoperative stay (days)	1.8±1.3	1.9±1.8	—	0.7
Postoperative stay (days)	6.2±1.3	7.5±3.7	—	0.4
Age (years)	59.4±5.4	58.5±11.0	—	0.9
Number of underlying conditions	2.2±1.9	1.1±0.9	—	0.2
Duration of operation (min)	284±64	292±87	—	0.9
Duration of bypass (min)	119±38	128±44	—	0.7
Duration of aortic clamping (min)	67±43	70±27	—	0.8
Amount of blood reperfused (mL)	903±236	901±317	—	1.0
Cardiac index[b]	2.8±0.6	3.0±0.5	—	0.6
Duration of treatment (days)				
Stay in cardiac ICU	2.2±0.4	2.9±2.2	—	0.8
Swan Ganz catheter	1.8±0.4	2.2±1.0	—	0.6
Arterial line	2±0	2.3±1.0	—	0.6
Mediastinal drains	2±0	2.2±0.8	—	0.6
Pacer wires	4.8±0.4	5.0±1.6	—	0.8
Ventilation	1±0	1.6±2.7	—	0.6
Antimicrobial prophylaxis	4.2±2.2	3.7±1.0	—	0.9

[a]Plus-minus values are means ±SD. NC denotes not calculable; ICU, intensive care unit.
[b]Cardiac index was defined as cardiac output in liters per minute per square meter of body surface area.
Source: Richet et al. (1991).[20]

bath provided the mechanism for the organism to be spread from nurse A's hands to the sterile field. Because nurse A was epidemiologically implicated in the investigation, cultures were obtained from a variety of sources highly likely to yield positive results. Culturing of the operating room environment and other personnel earlier in the investigation would have been unfocused, increasing the workload on the laboratory without significantly aiding the investigation.

Plan a More Systematic Study

Once a source and mode of transmission have been determined and you are able to make specific recommendations for control of the outbreak, you may want to perform additional studies. For example, after establishing by a case-control study that a certain group is at risk (e.g., hematology-oncology patients at risk for bacteremia), you may want to analyze that group further for other risk factors by using a cohort study model (e.g., to analyze duration of chemotherapy, specific chemotherapeutic agents, or duration of neutropenia). Serosurveys of patients and/ or HCWs can be performed to further define the population at risk after outbreaks of hepatitis B virus or anaphylactic reactions to certain drugs or products.

Evaluations of the efficacy of control measures that may have been undertaken before or during the investigation and of recommendations that the field team makes to the hospital can also be conducted at a later date.

Prepare a Written Report

Before departing from the field site, you should hold a meeting with staff of the health care facility and local or state health department representatives to apprise them of what you did and your results. The health care facility director and personnel are primarily interested in your recommendations for control measures. In fact, the legal department may ask you for recommendations from the first day of the investigation. As described earlier in this chapter, you can give preliminary recommendations based on previously documented guidelines for isolation, handwashing, and hospital environmental control and offer disease-specific prevention guidelines[21–27] at the beginning of or during the investigation. Additional recommendations based on your epidemiologic and laboratory data can be related to the facility at this debriefing. Your written report should describe any of the interim measures that were initiated and your final recommendations to the facility.

The written report for the facility, the state and local health department, and your supervisor should describe the problem as it was presented to you, the background information that you collected before and during the investigation, the methods and results of your investigation, and your final recommendations to the facility. The written report provides documentation of your investigation and therefore should accurately describe your actions. It is often helpful to write the report as you do the investigation. For example, write the background information before you arrive at the outbreak site, document your methods as you decide each step of the process (this is extremely important for case definitions, which may change during the course of the investigation), and compile a file of results as they become available (see Chapter 4). At your departure, you should be able to leave a brief written report that includes your recommendations for control measures with health care facility personnel. This report should be clearly marked as a *preliminary* document, as it will become part of the permanent record that can be used in court. After returning to your home office, a final report with "clean" data, final laboratory results, and more sophisticated statistical analysis can be written.

Medicolegal Aspects

Outbreaks of disease in health care facilities may lead to litigation against the facility. *Resist* all attempts by the facility administration to force you into making recommendations that your evidence and other relevant scientific data do not support. In addition, do not get caught up in interdepartmental politics and make recommendations without supporting data. A request for assistance in investigating an outbreak lends the health care facility an excellent defense in court, especially if recommended control measures were instituted and the problem brought under control.

Confidentiality laws and medical malpractice laws vary from state to state; conduct your investigation so that the confidentiality of patients and employees is ensured (see also Chapter 14). Therefore, you should not collect any identifying data that are not absolutely essential; if you must collect some kind of identifying data to link records, a convenient method is the hospital identification number (if it differs from the patient's social security number) or the patient's birth date and the last four digits of the social security number. If possible, put this information on your data collection form where it can easily be removed with a paper cutter (i.e., the top right-hand corner of the first page). This will also allow you to remove identifying data easily months later if a request for your information is made by a litigant. Under the Freedom of Information Act, patient or HCW names *cannot* be released by U.S. government workers.

SUMMARY

In summary, investigating outbreaks of disease in health care facilities is both similar to and different from investigating outbreaks in community settings. Both types of investigation involve a sick, frightened population who want immediate answers and solutions to the problem. Health care facilities have the advantage of multiple types of on-site records and a built-in professional staff of HCWs, both of which are invaluable resources during an outbreak investigation. And health care facilities provide the opportunity to study many aspects of disease in a closed, fairly well controlled setting. Cases of disease in health care facilities involve patients with complex attributes, and multivariate analysis of data may have to be conducted to control for host and device-related risk factors. On the other hand, health care facilities have the disadvantage of a fairly stressful work environment due to the legal implications of outbreaks in the health care setting.

Each state health department has state-specific regulations with which health care facilities must comply. Also, CDC has published guidelines relevant to the control of many infectious diseases in health care facilities.[21-31] These guidelines are meant to be a framework for individual health care facility staff to use when writing policy and procedure manuals for the facility. The Office of Safety and Health Administration (OSHA) writes the federal law that mandates certain practices in health care facilities; many of these laws incorporate CDC guidelines. In addition, the CDC guidelines and OSHA regulations are references which should be used during the course of outbreak investigations in health care facilities.

REFERENCES

1. Haley, R. W., Culver, D. H., White, J. W., et al. (1985). The nationwide nosocomial infection rate. *American Journal of Epidemiology*, 121, 159–67.
2. Cross, A. S., Roup, B. (1981). Role of respiratory assistance devices in endemic nosocomial pneumonia. *American Journal of Medicine*, 70, 681–85.
3. Haley, R. W., Culver, D. H., White, J. W., et al. (1985). The efficacy of infection surveillance and control programs in preventing nosocomial infections in U.S. hospitals. *American Journal of Epidemiology*, 121, 182–205.
4. Haley, R. W., Tenney, J. H., Lindsey, J. O. II, et al. (1985). How frequent are outbreaks of nosocomial infection in community hospitals? *Infection Control*, 6, 233–36.
5. Beck-Sague, C. M., Jarvis, W. R., Bland, L. A., et al. (1990). Outbreak of gram-negative bacteremia and pyrogenic reactions in a hemodialysis center. *American Journal of Nephrology*, 10, 397–403.
6. Jarvis, W. R. and the Epidemiology Branch, Hospital Infections Program (1991). Nosocomial outbreaks: The Centers for Disease Control's Hospital Infections Program experience, 1980–1990. *American Journal of Medicine*, 91(suppl 3B), 101S–106S.
7. Pegues, D. A., Shireley, L. A., Riddle, C. F., et al. (1991). *Serratia marcescens* surgical wound infection following breast reconstruction. *American Journal of Medicine*, 91(suppl 3B), 173S–78S.
8. Beck-Sague, C., Dooley, S. W., Hutton, M. D., et al. (1992). Hospital outbreak of multidrug-resistant *Mycobacterium tuberculosis* infections: Factors in transmission to staff and HIV-infected patients. *Journal of the American Medical Association*, 268, 1280–86.

9. Pearson, M. L., Jereb, J. A., Frieden, T. R., et al. (1992). Nosocomial transmission of multidrug-resistant *Mycobacterium tuberculosis:* A risk to patients and health care workers. *Annals of Internal Medicine,* 117, 191–96.

10. Edlin, B. R., Tokars, J. I., Grieco, M. H., et al. (1992). An outbreak of multidrug-resistant tuberculosis among hospitalized patients with the acquired immunodeficiency syndrome. *New England Journal of Medicine,* 326, 1514–21.

11. Centers for Disease Control and Prevention (1991). Anaphylactic reactions during general anesthesia among pediatric patients—United States, January 1990–January 1991. *Morbidity and Mortality Weekly Report,* 40, 437, 443.

12. Joint Commission on Accreditation of Healthcare Organizations (1990). Standards: Infection control. In *JCAHO, accreditation manual for hospitals.* Joint Commission on Accreditation of Healthcare Organizations, Chicago.

13. Garner, J. S., Jarvis, W. R., Emori, T. G., et al. (1988). CDC definitions for nosocomial infections, 1988. *American Journal of Infection Control,* 16, 128–40.

14. Knaus, W. A., Draper, E. A., Wagner, D. P., Zimmerman, J. E. (1985). APACHE II: A severity of disease classification system. *Critical Care Medicine,* 13, 818–29.

15. Pollack, M. M., Ruttimann, U. E, Getson, P. R. (1988). Pediatric risk of mortality (PRISM) score. *Critical Care Medicine,* 16, 1110–16.

16. Culver, D. H., Horan, T. C., Gaynes, R. P., et al. (1991). Surgical wound infection rates by wound class, operative procedure, and patient risk index. *American Journal of Medicine,* 91(suppl 3B), 152S–57S.

17. Gordon, S. M., Oshiro, L. S., Jarvis, W. R., et al. (1990). Foodborne snow mountain agent gastroenteritis with secondary person-to-person spread in a retirement community. *American Journal of Epidemiology,* 131, 702–10.

18. Beck-Sague, C. M., Jarvis, W. R., Brook, J. H., et al. (1990). Epidemic bacteremia due to *Acinetobacter baumannii* in five intensive care units. *American Journal of Epidemiology,* 132, 723–33.

19. Centers for Disease Control and Prevention (1990). Nosocomial transmission of multidrug-resistant tuberculosis to health-care workers and HIV-infected patients in an urban hospital—Florida. *Morbidity and Mortality Weekly Report,* 39, 718–22.

20. Richet, H. M., Craven, P. C., Brown, J. M., et al. (1991). A cluster of *Rhodococcus (Gordona) bronchialis* sternal-wound infections after coronary-artery bypass surgery. *New England Journal of Medicine,* 324, 104–9.

21. Garner, J. S., Favero, M. S. (1986). Guideline for handwashing and hospital environmental control. *American Journal of Infection Control,* 14, 110–29.

22. Simmons, B. P., Hooton, T. M., Wong, E. S., Allen, J. R. (1982). Guideline for prevention of intravascular infections. *Infection Control,* 3, 61–72.

23. Garner, J. S. (1986). Guideline for prevention of surgical wound infections. *American Journal of Infection Control,* 14, 71–80.

24. Wong, E. S., Hooton, T. M. (1983). Guideline for prevention of catheter-associated urinary tract infections. *American Journal of Infection Control,* 11, 28–33.

25. Simmons, B. P., Wong, E. S. (1982). Guideline for prevention of nosocomial pneumonia. *Infection Control,* 3, 327–33.

26. Garner, J. S., Simmons, B. P. (1983). Guideline for isolation precautions in hospitals. *Infection Control,* 4, 245–325.

27. Williams, W. W. (1983). Guideline for infection control in hospital personnel. *Infection Control* 4, 326–49.

28. Centers for Disease Control and Prevention (1991). Recommendations for prevent-

ing transmission of human immunodeficiency virus and hepatitis B virus to patients during exposure-prone invasive procedures. *Morbidity and Mortality Weekly Report*, 40(RR-8), 1–9.

29. Centers for Disease Control and Prevention (1990). Protection against viral hepatitis: Recommendations of the Immunization Practices Advisory Committee (ACIP). *Morbidity and Mortality Weekly Report*, 39(RR-2), 1–27.
30. Centers for Disease Control (1987). Recommendations for prevention of HIV transmission in health-care settings. *Morbidity and Mortality Weekly Report*, 36(2S), 3–18.
31. Centers for Disease Control and Prevention (1990). Guidelines for preventing the transmission of tuberculosis in health-care settings, with special focus on HIV-related issues. *Morbidity and Mortality Weekly Report*, 39(RR-17), 1–29.

16

INVESTIGATIONS IN CHILD CARE FACILITIES

Jacquelyn A. Polder
Janet Mohle-Boetani

An estimated 14 million children in the United States spend at least 10 hours per week in child care. Currently, 50 percent of mothers of children under the age of 1 year are employed outside the home; by the year 2000, a projected 75 percent of women with children under the age of 6 will be employed outside the home.[1] Because such a large and growing proportion of children spend extended periods of time in child care facilities (CCF), these settings have become an important epidemiologic entity within the community. Infectious diseases acquired in the community may spread rapidly among children and staff in CCFs and can then be transmitted further into the community. Both infectious disease and toxic exposures have resulted in outbreaks in day care programs; acute rather than chronic conditions are most often investigated.

This chapter attempts (1) to give the field investigator an understanding of the distinctive milieu and typical problems encountered during epidemic investigations of acute infectious disease problems in child care environments and (2) to provide a reference for conducting an investigation and implementing control efforts. The chapter focuses on communicable disease outbreaks and the operational aspects of their investigation, with only brief reference to descriptive and analytic analyses.

BACKGROUND CONSIDERATIONS

Recognizing and Reporting an Epidemic

Several factors unique to CCFs pose a challenge to public health in recognizing the occurrence of an outbreak, controlling spread of disease, and effectively intervening to prevent future outbreaks.

Child care programs may not keep daily health records on children in their programs. Although they may observe and report abnormalities to parents, they may not record symptoms or reasons for absences on a facility record. Moreover, children do not necessarily attend each day of the week. Some children attend only mornings or afternoons, and their signs and symptoms may not be noted by the staff. Thus, data regarding the health status of children in CCFs are usually not available or are incomplete.

Also, outbreaks may not be brought to the attention of public health authorities promptly because there may be no well-defined or well-understood system within the CCF for reporting disease or consulting with local health departments. In general, CCFs have no well-established connections to their local health departments.

Equally important, many outbreaks of infectious disease in CCFs present initially as a single case or as clusters of symptomatic illness without a definitive diagnosis (e.g., diarrhea, sore throat, rash, or vomiting). Because many of these signs and symptoms occur regularly in this setting, child care providers may not recognize outbreaks and may not seek outside medical advice. The staff may not request help until there is an easily detectable increase in incidence or severity of illness—for example, if more than 50 percent of the children are affected, an outbreak appears out of control, or a single child is hospitalized or diagnosed by a physician. By that time there may have been widespread transmission to families, siblings, friends, and other contacts of children in the CCF.

For local health departments, the recognition of an epidemic within a single CCF may be difficult, especially in large metropolitan areas where children come from a variety of backgrounds and geographic locations. A cluster of cases of a particular illness in one CCF may go undetected unless good communication and information sharing is routine among the health departments serving the different geographic areas where these children live.

In addition, because most health departments in the United States are struggling to maintain basic public health services due to increasing fiscal constraints, they may not have the financial or personnel support to maintain health department–initiated relationships with CCFs. In addition, health departments may not have the resources to recognize and respond to requests for consultation by child care providers.

Notification of outbreaks and requests for assistance may come from CCF directors. However, epidemics usually come to the attention of public health authorities when a physician or an upset parent reports directly to the local health department an illness in a child who attends a CCF. Sometimes, even the local media may report an unusual number or of ill children or an unusual type of illness.

THE INVESTIGATION

The steps of the investigation will follow those previously described (see Chapter 5), but especially as they relate to CCFs. Consideration will be given to the nature of children's exposures, the not infrequent widespread transmission to the community, and control measures particular to the CCF setting. However, before describing these steps, some unique epidemiologic aspects of the CCF need emphasis.

Outbreaks in CCFs may be difficult to recognize because the clinical presentations in children may vary from those seen in adults. Children often respond differently to exposures to organisms than do adults, and there may be several clinical expressions for any given infection. Investigations in child care facilities often have distinct and recurrent patterns. Outbreaks of infectious diseases in CCFs can be categorized in 4 groups[2]:

1. Infections that are spread among children in CCFs and that usually cause clinical illness in the children, providers, and older contacts. Shigellosis may spread rapidly both within CCFs and in secondary contacts of the children. The secondary transmission rate of shigellosis from a child to family members is estimated to be about 25 percent. Secondary transmission of rotavirus infection is estimated at 40 to 50 percent.

2. Organisms that spread between children who remain asymptomatic or only mildly symptomatic but cause recognizable clinical illness in their older contacts (i.e., siblings and parents). Community outbreaks of hepatitis A and giardiasis have been traced to children who have common child care associations. Hepatitis A in adults has been traced so often to children in CCFs that it is now recommended that if several adults with hepatitis have children at the same CCF, that CCF be considered the place of exposure until proved otherwise.[3] Two outbreaks of viral meningitis among adults caused by echovirus 30 were epidemiologically linked to their own children who attended common child care centers.[4,5] Because children may be asymptomatic yet can spread disease to older family members who develop symptoms, local health departments should review and investigate certain reported communicable diseases to determine a possible CCF association.

3. Illnesses that are easily spread in the child care setting, that do not frequently cause clinically evident illness in children or adults, but that may affect fetuses if contracted by pregnant women. Cytomegalovirus (CMV), rubella virus, and parvovirus B19 ("fifth disease") are examples of the more common organisms that may cause complications in susceptible pregnant women. Because these organisms may be commonly present and easily spread in CCFs and because young women of childbearing age frequently work in these settings, the consequences of such exposures should be considered as serious but preventable medical outcomes.

4. Organisms that are carried asymptomatically and spread between children but do not commonly cause clinical illness. For example, *Haemophilus influenzae* type b or *Neisseria meningitides* can be carried in the nasopharynx of many children in CCFs, but clinical illness is rare.[6] An investigation of a CCF with a child who died from group A streptococcal septicemia showed that 38 percent of his classmates carried the same strain of *Streptococcus* as the child but had no or only mild symptoms.[7]

Last, although no firm data are available regarding the true incidence of outbreaks of infectious disease in the CCF setting, organisms frequently identified in this setting include the following:

1. Bacteria
   - *Salmonella* and *Shigella* (fecal-oral spread)
   - *Haemophilus influenzae* (respiratory spread)
   - *Streptococcus* pharyngitis (respiratory spread)
2. Viruses
   - Rhinoviruses and other upper respiratory viruses (respiratory spread)
   - Norwalk agent, enterovirus, and other species causing gastroenteritis (fecal-oral and possibly respiratory spread).
   - Hepatitis A (fecal-oral spread)
3. Parasites
   - *Giardia* (fecal-oral spread)

Determine the Existence of an Outbreak

Child care programs do not routinely keep records of symptoms of children under their care. While they may inspect children daily and report findings to parents, they may not record symptoms or record reasons for absences. Thus a verbal report from the program director or parents may be the only evidence readily available for deciding if an outbreak truly exists. Child care facilities usually keep attendance records and records of medication administration; these data can be useful in evaluating the existence of an outbreak. If the diagnosis is not yet known, this preliminary information may assist in formulating a hypothesis regarding the infecting agent.

The local health department will usually have the most up-to-date numbers of cases that have been reported and the expected number of cases. However, you may need to verify these data by interviewing physicians or laboratory personnel or by reviewing clinic or laboratory data.

Confirm the Diagnosis

Review all known or suspected cases to determine whether any have sought medical advice and received a definitive diagnosis. Surveillance of local laboratory records may also yield additional information regarding trends in numbers of isolated pathogens. Recall that a handful of laboratory-confirmed cases (perhaps 8 to 12, depending upon the size of the outbreak) will usually be quite adequate for reasonable confirmation and continued investigation. However, rapid and proper collection of specimens can be difficult.

Since children are too young to provide consent for specimen collection, their parents must be contacted to give consent. This can be time-consuming and may create anxiety in parents and providers. If specimens must be collected, they should be collected by health department staff or members of the investigative team. While the CCF can be a convenient place for staff or parents to deposit laboratory specimens, the use of program space can be disruptive to the activities of the center. Unless closure of the CCF is indicated, the program should continue uninterrupted as much as possible. If specimens are collected, to avoid an association between discomfort and the child care setting, children should be examined and specimens collected in a room not used by the children under normal circumstances. The director's office and the staff break room have served well in some investigations.

If specimen collection or handling is done at several sites (private offices, emergency rooms, or at home), proper technique cannot be guaranteed, and this must be taken into consideration in the analysis. Some parents will not want to cooperate with the investigators but will take their child to a private physician for specimen collection. To educate the physicians regarding the outbreak and proper specimen collection, you will need to work closely with the local health network— including the health department, medical society, and possibly the media—to inform them about the nature of the problem, how to report cases, what specimens are needed, and how to collect them. If possible, visit whatever laboratories may be involved and confirm the diagnosis yourself.

Define a Case, Develop a Questionnaire, and Count Cases

Based on intensive interviewing of typical cases, develop a case definition to identify confirmed, presumptive, and possible cases. The definition should include a
composite of simple, objective, easily obtainable signs, symptoms, laboratory tests,
outcomes, or other epidemiologic characteristics.

As stated earlier, mere counting of cases is not enough. Since each situation
is unique, you will have to create a data collection instrument, to apply to each
case, that includes clinical, epidemiologic, and laboratory information pertinent
to the specific CCF setting.

It may be extremely important to observe and record how day care personnel perform their duties and how the children are handled. Questions specific to
the suspected agent should be collected (e.g., questions about food consumption
if a food-borne pathogen is suspected). But in addition, details regarding day-to-
day interactions of children within the child care setting will have to be collected.
For each case, classroom of primary attendance, hours at the center, movement in
the facility, contact with other children and staff, and whether the child wears
diapers at the center or at home should be collected. Larger child care centers may
have complex interactions between staff and children. Children may be primarily
cared for in small groups but may interact with other children in different classes
at various times of the day (e.g., on the playground, at lunch or snack time, in art
activities, or on field trips). Staff may work primarily with one group of children
but rotate periodically to different groups, as during rest periods or meals. Patterns and hours of attendance of children at the center may vary as well. Often,
school-age children are in attendance in the early morning and late afternoon; they
may mingle with the younger children.

Understanding the patterns of movement and activity among children will
enhance recognition of common exposures among cases and contribute to the
development of a hypothesis for the cause of the outbreak.

After creating the questionnaire, identify as many cases within the CCF as
possible. If person-to-person spread is suspected, find the close contacts of cases.
The number of contacts will depend upon class size and cohorting policies. There
are clearly many possible combinations of child care and staff rotations. For example, in some centers, children are cared for in groups of three to five children
of similar age. In other programs, many children of all ages interact with each
other. Groups of children are often cared for together in the morning and then in
the late afternoon, as well as during special activities such as art work and outside
play.

Unlike investigations in many other settings, investigation of child–care associated outbreaks and the search for additional cases may involve more extensive review of community cases. Children in CCFs also interact closely with fam-

ily, friends, and community contacts outside of child care. Therefore, you may need to search the child's family and other contacts for additional primary or secondary cases. Contacts of cases should also be identified to determine potential exposures and contacts who may need prophylaxis.

Active surveillance for cases can be arranged through local emergency clinics, physicians' offices, or other appropriate settings. Recognize that there is virtually no routine surveillance for acute or chronic disease in CCF.

Finding and evaluating cases by phone calls or visits to health care providers, other child care providers, hospitals, parents, or others involved in the care of the cases can be time-consuming. Child care staff are usually very concerned about the occurrence of illness in their attendees and its possible association with their center. They may be reluctant to share the names and phone numbers of parents and children in their care. Personnel of the CCF will have to be assured of the need to investigate to prevent additional cases and that confidentiality will be maintained. In addition, even after having obtained names and phone numbers from the child care staff, the task of finding parents may be time-consuming, because most will be away from home during the day and may not be reachable at their places of employment. Telephoning parents may be most productive in the early evening hours.

The investigation should include many visits to the involved CCF. These visits will include interviews with the director or owner/operator and persons providing hands-on care of children. These are stressful times for the staff, and reassurance will be necessary to ensure cooperation with the investigating team. Because these are time-intensive visits, 1/2 to 1 day per visit may be required.

Orient the Data According to Time, Place, and Person

As with all field investigations, this is the time to organize your descriptive data into a logical time, place, and person relationship (see Chapter 6). Information like that described above will have to be analyzed, particularly data relating to (1) the hours a child spends at the center (both the number and the specific hours), or, if the cases include parents, the hours their children spend in the program; (2) whether the child wears diapers in the CCF or at home (enteric diseases like hepatitis A are spread more widely in centers that care for children with diapers[8] (3) the groups of children with whom the ill child interacts; and (4) in a possible food-borne outbreak, the source (home and/or CCF) of food and snacks.

Determine Who Is at Risk

With properly drawn epidemic curves—often including epidemic-associated cases and non-epidemic-associated cases—the critical times of transmission and exposure can be deduced. Spot maps such as those showing playrooms with and without infected children can be extremely useful in drawing useful inferences. After integration of time and place with the unique traits of the ill children, a clear epidemiologic picture of who is at risk should emerge.

Develop and Test a Hypothesis

After the population at risk has been defined, a plausible scenario of events that fits with the known facts and the epidemiology of the confirmed or presumed agent should be developed. In most instances, analyses will be case-control studies where comparisons will be made between ill children and similar but healthy controls in regard to possible unique exposures. Some CCFs have written menus (including snacks) that make finding exposures associated with food-borne outbreaks much easier. If children are routinely placed in well-defined groups, then a cohort study may be the easiest way to analyze the data. However, children frequently intermingle with one another in CCFs, and defining exposed versus unexposed groups may be difficult. In one investigation of giardiasis, careful interviewing about specific activities and how children interacted throughout the day led the field team to implicate "wading pool parties" as a risk factor for the transmission of *Giardia*.[9]

Transmission of infection from children to their household contacts may involve certain risk factors identifiable by investigating particular behaviors between contacts and the child. For example, in two outbreaks of viral meningitis among parents of children attending a child care center, adults who usually washed their hands after changing diapers were less likely to become infected than adults who reported less frequent handwashing.[4,5]

If several child care programs appear to be experiencing similar outbreaks and appropriate centers can be identified as controls for the analysis, one may be able to identify center characteristics that are risk factors for transmission. Investigation of a multicenter outbreak of shigellosis in Lexington, Kentucky, found that outbreaks of shigellosis occurred more often in centers where employees not only changed diapers but served food to the children as well.[10]

Plan a More Systematic Study

After the outbreak has been controlled, some CCFs may agree to participate in a more extensive study. Getting cooperation may be directly related to the cooperation developed and the performance of the field team during the investigation. But even very cooperative directors or owners may decline to participate. Child care facilities are often understaffed, and even the monitoring of seemingly simple logistical details may prove to be too costly. Answering an additional questionnaire may be viewed by staff and parents as too time-consuming. They also may not want their children to experience the discomfort entailed in further investigations. Recently developed techniques to analyze blood from finger-sticks and saliva may make studies in CCFs easier in the future. As always, questionnaires should be kept as simple and short as possible.

Prepare a Written Report

In addition to preparing a report for local health officials, consider sharing the findings with the CCF and interested parents. This report can serve several purposes. In the early stages of the investigation, the promise of a written document can be used to promote cooperation with the study. A preliminary summary can encourage participation in any additional investigations that may be needed.

The final report should be written in lay terms and should reinforce control measures if needed. A report provides the CCF staff and parents with tangible evidence of the study they contributed to and encourages their participation in the future.

Execute Control and Prevention Measures

Early in the investigation, often before laboratory confirmation is obtained, general control measures can be started. For example, person-to-person spread of most organisms can be greatly reduced by reinforcement of appropriate handwashing techniques; that is, handwashing after toileting activities, including diaper changes, and before food handling or activities involving hand-to-mouth exposure (e.g., eating, smoking, or applying makeup). Handwashing after contact with saliva or respiratory secretions and careful cleaning of children's toys may reduce transmission of respiratory tract infections or other diseases transmitted by oral/fecal contact. Other control measures include excluding children with diarrhea from the CCF, caring for children strictly in small groups, separating diaper changing and food preparation areas, monitoring of handwashing, and handwashing upon arrival at the child care center by both children and staff.

In addition to the general control measures referred to above, more specific measures can be instituted once either the diagnosis is confirmed or risk factors are clearly evident. For example, after confirming the diagnosis of meningococcal meningitis, rifampin may be given to classmates and close contacts of an ill child.

Be sure to work closely with the proper health officials in making further recommendations. This will likely be an ongoing process. Update the child care staff immediately regarding these changes and the rationale behind them. Daily surveillance should be established, so that any additional cases will be reported regularly to all concerned and control efforts can be monitored. Even after control has been gained, active surveillance should be continued, probably for several weeks or months.

Routine recommendations regarding exclusion of children from CCFs and environmental modifications may have to be adjusted based on the severity and magnitude of the outbreak, local regulations, and publicity surrounding the situation. For example, some diseases—such as shigellosis, salmonellosis, giardiasis, and *Escherichia coli* 0157: H7 infections—would normally require exclusion from a CCF.[11] However, if there are large numbers of children with active disease, cohorting should be considered.[12] This alternative would allow children to attend designated CCFs and permit parents to remain on the job.

Child care providers are generally not trained health professionals. Although, after some experience, they can usually recognize common childhood diseases such as chickenpox or measles, they should not be expected to diagnose or assess the severity of illnesses. But child care staff should be trained to recognize symptoms and signs in children that may require immediate medical attention and exclusion from the CCF. They should understand when it is important for them to report an illness to their superiors and the local health department.

Furthermore, during an epidemic investigation, the providers may feel threatened by the epidemiologist; the staff may feel that they are at fault, that their CCF may receive negative publicity, and that parents will withdraw their children from the CCF. Cooperation will be facilitated by considering these possible anxieties and reassuring the providers.

Many child care providers and parents of children in child care do not have comprehensive health insurance or adequate leave or vacation time to stay home when either they or their children are sick. Thus, child care staff may remain on the job and children may be left at CCFs while they are ill. These become critical factors in potential control of disease both within the outbreak setting and elsewhere in other CCFs. When children are prevented from attending a CCF, parents may be forced to seek alternative care, often in a site that accepts "drop-ins." This practice may inadvertently expose a new group of susceptible children and staff and continue the outbreak in a new setting. Control of highly infectious or serious conditions may include recommendations that local health department staff contact all parents of excluded children on a daily basis to ensure compliance.

Last, local health departments frequently do not have personnel specifically dedicated to understanding and reviewing the needs of CCFs, evaluating their problems, and providing ongoing consultation to them. An outbreak may be the only contact the CCF will have with the local health department. Therefore, health department personnel may have to be educated regarding the concerns and operation of CCFs in order to carry out investigations most effectively and apply the necessary control efforts.

SUMMARY

The primary purposes of conducting an outbreak investigation in a child care setting are to identify the cause of the outbreak, interrupt continued spread, and make recommendations for future prevention of disease. Because of the uniqueness of the child care setting, field investigations may be challenging. Recognition of epidemics in CCFs is often difficult and delayed because of inexperienced staff, few or no internal standards of record keeping or reporting, and lack of good communication with local health departments. Control efforts are hampered because of multiple interactions between CCF children, staff, and their families. However, close collaboration between CCF personnel, local health authorities, and the field team can usually control and prevent epidemics in CCFs by careful application of epidemiologic methods, simple hygienic practices, health education, and improved reporting practices.

REFERENCES

1. Dawson, D. A., and Cain, V. S. (1990). *Child care arrangements: Health of our nation's children, United States, 1988. Advance data from vital statistics, no. 187.* National Center for Health Statistics, Hyattsville, Maryland.
2. Goodman, R. A., Osterholm, M. T., Granoff, D. M., Pickering L. K. (1994). Infectious diseases and child care. *Journal of Pediatrics*, 74, 134–9.
3. Shapiro, C. N., Hadler, S. C. (1991). Hepatitis A and hepatitis B virus infections in the day care setting. *Pediatric Annals*, 20(8), 435–36, 438–41.
4. Helfand, R., Khan, A., Pallansch, M., et al. (1994). Echovirus 30 infection and aseptic meningitis in parents of children attending a child care center. *Journal of Infectious Disease*, 169:1133–37.
5. Mohle-Boetani, J., Matkin, C., Pallansch, M. et al. Echovirus 30 outbreak in a child care center: Risk factors for transmission from children to parents. [Abstract #1425.] Presented at the 33rd Interscience Conference on Antimicrobial Agents and Chemotherapy, October 17–20, 1993, New Orleans, Louisiana.
6. Murphy, T. V., Granoff, D., Chrane, D. F., et al. (1985). Pharyngeal colonization with *Haemophilus influenzae* type b in children in a day care center without invasive disease. *Journal of Pediatrics*, 106, 712–16.
7. Engelgau, M. M., Woernle, C., Schwartz, B., et al. (1994). Group A streptococcal carriage in an Alabama day care center following a fatal invasive case. *Proceedings of the International Conference on Child Care Health: Science, Prevention, and Practice. Pediatrics*, 94(6), 1030.
8. Hadler, S. C., Erben, J. J., Francis, D. P., et al. (1982). Risk factors for hepatitis A in day care center. *Journal of Infectious Diseases*, 145, 255–61.
9. Moore, A. C., Finton, R. J., Kreckman, L. A., et al. (1992). Outbreaks of giardiasis in two day care centers: Evidence of transmission through wading pools. [Abstract.] Presented at the International Conference on Child Day Care Health: Science, Prevention, and Practice, June 15, 1992, Atlanta, Georgia.

10. Mohle-Boetani, J. M., Stapleton, M, Finger, R., et al. (1995). Community-wide shigellosis: Control of an outbreak and risk factors in child day-care centers. *American Journal of Public Health*, 95(6):812–16.
11. Belongia, E. A., Osterholm, M. T., Solar, J. T., et al. (1993). Transmission of *Escherichia coli* O157:H7 infection in Minnesota child day-care facilities. *The Journal of the American Medical Association*, 269, 883–88.
12. Tauxe, R. V., Johnson, K. E., Boase, J. C., et al. (1986). Control of day care shigellosis: A trial of convalescent day care in isolation. *American Journal of Public Health*, 75, 627–30.

17

EPIDEMIOLOGIC INVESTIGATIONS
IN INTERNATIONAL SETTINGS

Stanley O. Foster

Envision yourself assigned to investigate an epidemic of an unknown disease in an unfamiliar area of the world and in a country where both the language and culture are different from anything you have previously experienced. Such an assignment encapsulates the challenge of international epidemiology. Although the approach to international field investigations is similar to the approach described in Chapter 5, this chapter emphasizes some of the unique aspects of carrying out an investigation in an international setting.

GETTING READY

Most requests for epidemiologic assistance arise from adverse health events brought to the government's attention through the press or political system. Outbreaks are generally of two types: (1) large outbreaks of a major epidemic disease (yellow fever, cholera, meningococcal meningitis) or (2) acute episodes of unexplained mortality such as those caused by adulterated drugs or foods, toxic exposures, or rare hemorrhagic fevers. Detection is often delayed because of poor morbidity and mortality surveillance, the frequent occurrence of these events in remote rural areas, and the tendency of officials to overlook potential problems in the hope that they will disappear. When the outbreaks do become public, there is often a sense of panic. For the public health official pressured to act, the arrival of technical assistance provides a visible sign of government response to the emergency. The request frequently carries the expectation of external resources to control the problem.

When you receive a request from a national health authority, it is important that you immediately acknowledge receipt and identify a time frame within which a response will be forthcoming. You should contact the World Health Organization (WHO), international and bilateral agencies working in the country, and the diplomatic mission to which you will be attached. These early contacts are useful in verifying the need for epidemiologic assistance, providing additional information on the outbreak, identifying other ongoing requests for assistance, and, most importantly, opening the channels of communication for in-country collaboration and support.

The typically short lead time between receipt of a request and departure (hours to days) requires that you prepare carefully. Place a high priority on arranging travel (some countries have only one flight in and out per week) and obtaining a visa or visas. The latter will require a current passport, passport photos, and contact with the diplomatic mission accredited to grant visas. Clearances on the provision of technical assistance, preferably in writing, should be obtained from the requesting country, the funding agency, and your own supervisor (if you want to have a job when you return). Advance information on flight number and arrival time should be communicated to an in-country contact with a request for airport assistance. Airport assistance will frequently reduce the hassle of immigration and customs and is especially important when the investigation requires carrying a computer (restricted in many countries) or laboratory equipment.

Your personal health merits attention. Common health hazards can be identified by contacting experts in the health of travelers. Such experts are located at most larger health departments, major hospitals, and quarantine facilities. Written health guidelines for international travel are available from WHO and from many public health agencies. Immunization status must be assessed and brought up to date, including boosters for tetanus and polio. Travelers to areas where yellow fever is endemic will need a valid yellow fever certificate. All travelers who could potentially go to remote areas should obtain gamma globulin prophylaxis for hepatitis A. Travelers to malarious areas need to initiate appropriate chemoprophylaxis. If travel is to an area where *Plasmodium falciparum* is endemic and drug-resistant strains have been identified, a malaria expert should be contacted about current recommendations for chemoprophylaxis and backup disease treatment. As medical resources may be limited or of questionable quality in-country, you should assemble a basic medical kit for personal use that includes antipyretics, antihistamines, a broad-spectrum antibiotic, eye ointment, oral rehydration salts (ORS) for treatment of dehydrating diarrheas, water purification tablets, a thermometer, and simple bandages. Other important items to pack include a canteen, a flashlight with extra batteries, a Swiss Army–type knife, a hat, an extra pair of glasses, soap, towel, and plastic gloves (in case you are required to provide first aid). While sunglasses are useful during travel, they are, in some cultures, a barrier to effective communication. Clear glasses are recommended during interpersonal communications. Carry any prescription medicines and all essential items in your hand baggage in case your checked luggage is lost en route.

Consider your money and clothing needs carefully. Because credit cards and travelers' checks may not be accepted, cash may be needed. If it is possible that you will need to fund upcountry travel, gasoline, or field staff, establish a mechanism for transfer of funds. For personal safety reasons, carrying large amounts of cash is not recommended. Wear a money belt. Pack lightly. Include one suit for official visits; a few sets of hand-washable, comfortable clothes; good walking shoes; and sneakers. As investigations scheduled for a few weeks may on occasion last for months, set aside one evening before you leave for family or close friends.

As international investigations frequently involve unknown or unfamiliar conditions, use the few available hours to read up on possible disease etiologies, collect a few key references, identify potential backup technical expertise that will be available to respond if needed (e.g., epidemiologic, statistical, laboratory), and talk to individuals who have worked in the country.[1] Depending on the nature of the request, consider the need for clerical supplies, a portable computer, and specimen collection and shipping materials. Keep a diary of events, persons met, and data in a bound notebook (loose pieces of paper can be a disaster). Be sure that any electrical equipment is compatible in voltage and plug type to what is available at your destination. More than a few 110-volt computers have been ruined when they were plugged into a 220-volt line. Solar calculators are an excellent investment, both for work in remote villages without electricity and as a token of appreciation for collaborating field staff.

Perhaps the most important part of the preparation is the collection of one or two books on the country and culture for reading in transit. Cultural differences are significant and important.[2–4] In certain societies, it is inappropriate to shake hands with members of the opposite sex. In others, showing the sole of your shoe is a major breach of etiquette. Mistakes will be made, but a few small steps demonstrating good faith and affirming your recognition and appreciation of the new culture will facilitate the development of effective working relationships. Knowledge of a country's history, geography, and greetings in the local language is a good place to start.

THE FIRST DAY

The first day is important both in terms of whom you meet and the order in which you meet them. Critical to success is your attitude. Are you the "knight in shining armor" coming to solve an important problem, or a colleague coming to work with national authorities to help them solve their problem?[3] The latter approach is the only appropriate one. In many cultures it is necessary to establish rapport before proceeding with substantive discussions. Finding areas of common interest is an art that requires preparation and practice. During the protocol visits, assistance in identifying a responsible national to participate as a coinvestigator should be solicited. If you are not familiar with the language of the country, you may also need an interpreter. In recruiting an interpreter, be specific as to what you want—an individual willing to travel under difficult circumstances and for a long period of time. Be sure to finalize the terms of employment in writing as well as the source of funding.

Before heading to the field, collect information on what is already known about the outbreak: the affected area and the basic epidemiologic questions of who, what, when, and where. It is useful to determine how the outbreak came to public attention, the nature and timing of a response, and the reasons for the request. Be sure that you are providing the requested information and services.

Logistics is a major challenge for the field epidemiologist. Reliable transport, a driver, maps, gasoline, spare tire or tires, a jack, and a lug wrench often require time and frequently some ingenuity to obtain. Do not take the driver's word for it, check out the transport yourself. Take the time to discuss with the driver your expectations regarding his driving, such as obeying the speed limit and not passing on hills. Ensuring compliance, especially during the first hour of travel, is good prevention. A reliable driver is worth his weight in gold. When available, request a vehicle with seat belts. In many countries, it is dangerous to drive at night. If that is the case, do not do so. If safe water and food are not available in the affected area, these, too, must be procured. In areas where blood supplies are not properly screened, transfusions are dangerous.

THE INVESTIGATION

After many days of preparation, you will feel eager to get on with the investigation and examine cases. However, the prelude to any field investigation is the introduction to the local authorities. These visits should be viewed not as protocol but as team recruitment. Local authorities will serve as guides, provide introductions at the community and household levels, and facilitate community and family participation in the investigation. In addition, local authorities may have access to the only comfortable places to sleep and eat.

Once the existence of an epidemic has been established, the next step in the investigation is the establishment of a case definition. This will require collecting a clinical history and doing a physical examination on several, preferably recent cases. If timely laboratory support is not available, cases will usually be defined on clinical grounds. Where possible, use simple and workable definitions, such as those established by WHO. For example, the WHO case definition of polio-myelitis includes acute onset of asymmetrical flaccid paralysis without sensory change; that for neonatal tetanus includes death with spasms between days 5 and 15 days of life after a normal birth in which breast-feeding was established; and that for shigellosis is simply diarrhea with blood.

Once a case definition has been established, the next task is finding cases. Determining when and where cases occurred will frequently require the ingenu-ity and assistance of local political, religious, and traditional authorities. With a lay-adapted case definition and a list of geographic subunits (e.g., districts, vil-lages), the challenge is to find the quickest and cheapest way to identify cases. This may utilize telephone contact among local authorities, police radio contact, or the sending out of traditional messengers on foot. On some occasions, it may be necessary to organize an active community-to-community search. Such sur-veys must be well planned and involve several key steps: (1) the recruitment and selection of personnel, (2) the development and testing of the data collection in-strument, (3) on-the-job training of the staff in the field survey techniques, (4) utilization of field training to refine the survey instrument, and (5) the mobiliza-tion of logistic support (see Chapter 11).

The conduct of the investigation will require an understanding of cultural norms and practices. For example, in some Muslim cultures, where men are not allowed to enter a house or talk to women, enumerators will have to be female. In developing the survey instrument and carrying out interviews, knowledge of the local health belief model is useful. For individuals who traditionally attribute ill-ness to a curse or to the supernatural, biological causality does not make much sense.

Epidemiologists called to provide assistance often encounter events worthy of in-depth investigation and eventual publication. It is, however, important to give priority to the reasons for which your assistance was requested: the identifi-cation of etiology or the route of exposure or the establishment of control activities. Once an etiology is identified and control measures are agreed upon, control activities should become the primary focus of attention. Monitoring the quality and effectiveness of these control actions often requires new and creative approaches.

COMMUNICATING AND REPORTING

An important aspect of the investigation is keeping those who are responsible informed. This includes the officials who requested the investigation, local health officials, political or traditional leaders cooperating in the investigation, and technical experts at the investigator's home institution. In areas where telephones do not exist or do not function, alternative means of communication must be identified (e.g., police or shortwave radio). If communication is difficult, it is useful to set up a schedule for contact. Radio messages must be discretely worded to avoid misinterpretation by others with radio access. In some remote areas, couriers may be needed to transport messages via local transport or on foot.

Before leaving the country, the team has the responsibility to report on the investigative findings and the recommended actions, first to those responsible and additionally to others involved in the request or follow-up actions. While hand-prepared audiovisuals such as transparencies are often useful in making the presentation, handouts or flip charts provide backup in case of power failure. Prepare and distribute a written draft report. Results of the investigation must be clearly presented in a language understandable to the intended audience. Acknowledgement should be given to the individuals assisting in the investigation.

As indicated in several chapters of this book, there is one key rule regarding the role of the visiting epidemiologist and the press: requests for information should be referred to the appropriate national authority. On rare occasions, where national authorities request a briefing with the media, the interviews should be carried out jointly.

PUBLICATION

Where appropriate, publication must to be handled sensibly. Authorship, including at least one local collaborator, should be agreed to in advance. All articles need clearance in writing from the host country prior to publication.

MAINTAINING PERSPECTIVE

As a visiting epidemiologist, your salary may be fifty to a hundred times that of your national colleagues. Living and working in such a situation requires both wisdom and tact. Acceptance of hospitality from an impoverished village leader is difficult but necessary. As the leader's youngest children may go hungry when visitors are fed, a modest appetite is suggested. Small tokens of appreciation such as books or calculators are appropriate gifts. Except for drivers, monetary gifts are not recommended.

On your return home, thank you notes, technical publications, postcards, and picture books provide continuity to friendships that have developed.

SUMMARY

The opportunity to participate in epidemiologic investigations in cultures and countries other than your own is one of the challenges and rewards of epidemiology. During such investigations, you are a guest whose responsibility is to work with national colleagues in solving their problems. This chapter outlines a number of practical steps for the field epidemiologist: getting ready, the first day in the new country, carrying out the field investigation, and communicating results.

REFERENCES

1. Centers for Disease Control and Prevention (1992). Famine-affected, refugee, and displaced populations: Recommendations for public health issues. *Morbidity and Mortality Weekly Report*, 41 (RR-13), 1–76.
2. Brislin, R. W. (1982). *Cross-cultural encounters*. Pergamon Press, New York.
3. Allegra, D. T., Nieburg, P., Grabe, M. (eds.) (1984). *Emergency refugee health care— A chronicle of experience in the Khymer assistance operation, 1979–1980*. chaps 30–32; pp. 163–81. Centers for Disease Control, Atlanta.
4. Centers for Disease Control (1987). *Crossing cultures? Some suggestions to smooth the way*. Centers for Disease Control, Atlanta.

18

LABORATORY SUPPORT FOR THE
EPIDEMIOLOGIST IN THE FIELD

This chapter provides some general guidelines as to what specimens are appropriate to collect when you are investigating an infectious disease problem or studying a potential chemical toxic exposure. When you encounter an illness likely to be of infectious etiology, there is no substitute for good clinical judgment. Many of the laboratory tests discussed here provide information to support a diagnosis, not to make it. Additionally, the lists of specimens to be collected and tests to be performed are not exhaustive and may not include newer investigative or research tools such as genome probing. For the microbial agents, no effort was made to include all possible agents, only the more common ones.

The section on chemical toxicants, below, gives only general instructions on how to collect specimens. An example of the necessary detail and care required to collect certain kinds of specimens is also given to emphasize the critical nature of the methods used (see Appendix 18–2). Remember, these are general guidelines and are provided here mainly to begin to direct your attention to the kinds of

Thanks are due to William Martone, M.D., and David Bell, M.D., Hospital Infections Program, and other staff in the National Center for Infectious Diseases who provided much of the information in this Chapter. Thanks are also due to Jane Neese, Ph.D., former Chief, Special Activities Branch, John Liddle, Ph.D, Assistant Director for Emergency Response and State Programs, and Elaine Gunter, BS, MT(ASCP) Chief, NHANES Laboratory, Division of Environmental Health Laboratory Sciences, National Center for Environmental Health, who provided all the material relating to chemical toxins.

specimens that are appropriate for laboratory examination and the general precautions and instructions that are necessary for proper collection and storage. *As has been emphasized before, make early contact with your laboratory-scientist counterpart before collection.* Seek out the local, state, or provincial laboratory directors as appropriate. Many of these laboratories will perform many or most of the tests described below—particularly those relating to infectious diseases.

If, on the other hand, you are contemplating the collection and transport of specimens for chemical toxicant examination at CDC, it is imperative that you make contact with the National Center for Environmental Health (NCEH) laboratory before making the collection. This is absolutely essential, as NCEH has or will create detailed protocols for you. If there is an emergency, NCEH is on call and will send materials (kits) and instructions as soon as possible.

The National Center for Infectious Disease (NCID) will provide laboratory services to state health departments under special, clearly defined circumstances. You should be aware of a document entitled, *Reference and Disease Surveillance* printed by NCID in February 1993. This publication specifies the kinds of specimens that will be processed for state health departments, the kinds of tests that will be performed, and considerable detail regarding the collection and shipment of specimens to CDC. The NCID will not process specimens submitted to it from county health departments, hospitals, or private physicians. All specimens must be sent to the state health department laboratory initially. If the state laboratory subsequently deems it necessary to call upon the laboratories of NCID for support and if the specimens satisfy the CDC requirements, then the NCID laboratories will process the specimens.

COLLECTION OF SPECIMENS FOR POTENTIAL CHEMICAL TOXICANTS—GENERAL INSTRUCTIONS

For both regularly scheduled studies and emergency response, laboratory results are only as good as the specimens collected, regardless of how sophisticated the analytical method may be. Unlike specimens of biological agents for which collectors must protect themselves from exposure, specimens from cases of chemical toxicant exposure must frequently be protected from additional contamination by collectors. Extraneous substances from the ambient air or the collectors' skin or clothing, or interfering substances in the collection and storage supplies, will be concentrated and measured along with the specimens, yielding falsely elevated values.

In acute chemical exposures, most toxicants or their metabolites are rapidly cleared from easily accessible specimens such as blood, either through excretion or sequestration in tissues. The primary compounds or their metabolites may be quite unstable; therefore speed of response and prompt collection and shipment of specimens are critical factors.

In cases of suspected chemical toxicant exposure, it is extremely important to work in conjunction with the analytical support laboratory, or, if needed, with the Division of Environmental Health Laboratory Sciences, NCEH, CDC, to obtain correct information about proper specimen collection/processing/storage/shipment prior to analysis. Conditions vary greatly depending upon whether an organic or inorganic chemical toxicant is suspected, and unless specimens are properly prepared, achieving valid analytical data is impossible. Table 18–1 summarizes collection and storage procedures for chemical toxicant analyses recommended by CDC.

Types of different collection information to be considered include:

1. What is the correct specimen to collect? For recent exposures blood is often the most useful specimen. For longer term exposures or body burden urine may be the specimen of choice.
2. If blood, what type of Vacutainer/anticoagulant should be used?
3. If an inorganic trace element is suspected, Vacutainers and storage containers must be pre-screened by the laboratory to prevent background contamination of the specimen.
4. If a urine specimen is to be collected, is a preservative required?
5. Must samples be shipped refrigerated within 24 hours of collection, or can they be batched, frozen, and shipped on dry ice?
6. What volume of blood or urine is required?
7. Are tissue samples required (adipose or autopsy materials) for analysis rather than urine or blood?
8. Is the suspected toxicant a cholinesterase inhibitor (such as a pesticide or nerve gas)?
9. Is a suspected food source available?

In case of a true emergency such as an acute exposure, where time does not permit contacting the laboratory to obtain a proper protocol and collection supplies, a good rule of thumb is to obtain biological specimens (whole blood, serum, and urine) as soon as possible, even if it means using materials not pretested by the support laboratory. In these rare cases, remember the basic guidelines for controlling extraneous contamination and cooling the specimens as soon as possible to prevent degradation. To allow evaluation of possible extraneous contamination from the collection materials on hand, randomly select at least three of each container (such as Vacutainers, collection cups, storage vials), seal them in a clean container such as a large Ziplock bag, and ship them with the specimens to the support laboratory. However, you should obtain collection materials supplied by the support laboratory as soon as possible for all subsequent sampling.

Table 18–1. CDC-Recommended Specimen Collection Summary
for Possible Chemical Toxicants

SUSPECTED TOXICANT	PREFERRED SPECIMEN (IN DECREASING ORDER)	ADULTS AND CHILDREN (10 YEARS OLD AND OLDER)	BABIES AND CHILDREN (LESS THAN 10 YEARS OLD)
Organic	serum	2 10-mL silicone-free Vacutainers, freeze serum	1 10-mL silicone-free Vacutainer, freeze serum
	urine	50-100 mL in prescreened collection cup, store in 60-mL glass Wheaton bottle, freeze	25-100 mL in prescreened collection cup or pediatric collection bag, store in 60-mL glass Wheaton bottle, freeze
	whole blood (heparin for most analytes, gray-top for volatiles)	1-2 10 mL tubes, refrigerate	1 10-mL tube, refrigerate
Inorganic	urine	50-100 mL in prescreened collection cup (no preservative if frozen promptly)	25-100 mL in prescreened collection cup (no preservative if frozen promptly)
	whole blood (usually EDTA)	1 2-3 mL prescreened Vacutainer, refrigerate	1 2-3 mL prescreened Vacutainer, refrigerate
	serum	1 7-mL trace elements Vacutainer, freeze serum	1 7-mL trace elements Vacutainer, freeze serum
Unknown	serum	3 10-mL silicone-free Vacutainers, freeze serum	1 10-mL silicone-free Vacutainer, freeze serum
	urine	50-100 mL in prescreened collection cup, store in 60-mL glass Wheaton bottle, freeze	25-100 mL in prescreened collection cup, store in 60-mL glass Wheaton bottle, freeze
	whole blood, EDTA	1 2-3 mL prescreened Vacutainer, refrigerate	1 2-3 mL prescreened Vacutainer, refrigerate
	whole blood, heparin (especially if exposure to cholinesterase inhibitor suspected)	1 7-10 mL heparin Vacutainer, refrigerate	1 5-7 mL heparin Vacutainer, refrigerate
	tissues, autopsy materials, stomach contents	10-50 g, frozen, no preservative, seal in small Ziplock bag placed in plastic specimen container	10-50 g, frozen, no preservative, seal in small Ziplock bag placed in plastic specimen container
	food (as much of suspected material as available: place in large Ziplock bags, freeze if perishable)		

When requested by state and local laboratories, the Division of Environmental Health Laboratory Sciences (EHLS), NCEH, CDC, will provide laboratory support for environmental health studies and emergency response situations involving potential chemical toxicant exposures. As with other epidemiologic investigations, these studies must be planned and submitted for all appropriate processing as soon as possible. If any analyses are to be performed by EHLS, a detailed study protocol will be prepared to be included as an appendix in the study protocol. The EHLS laboratories maintain pretested specimen collection supplies and abbreviated collection instructions (by specimen type) that can be shipped by express courier, or prepared to accompany the investigator.

Materials Required for Specimen Collection

Available locally

The following materials must be supplied or be available locally by prior arrangement with a support laboratory:

1. Centrifuge capable of spinning 10-mL or 16- X 100-mm Vacutainer tubes at 1500 x G for 15 minutes
2. Refrigerator (4–8 °C) and non-frost free freezer (£ -20 °C)
3. Dry ice, 30–40 lb on hand (10–15 lb per shipping container), and insulated gloves for safely handling dry ice
4. General phlebotomy supplies, other than specific Vacutainer types, and biohazard disposal containers

Materials supplied by support laboratories

All other specimen collection/processing/shipment supplies should be provided by the support laboratory, with all materials identified in the protocol, for proper use.

All of these materials (Vacutainers, pipets, storage vials, etc.) will have been screened or specially washed and packaged to minimize extraneous contamination. USE ONLY THE MATERIALS SUPPLIED for specimens if they are to be sent to CDC, and do not open any packages until they are to be used. Return any unused supplies to the support laboratory.

Detailed instructions for collecting each specimen type should be included with the collection supplies. The protocol for packaging and shipping the specimens will also be attached. Examples of chemical toxicant specimen collection protocols for emergency situations are outlined in Table 18–2.

General Considerations to be Kept in Mind at All Times

Specimen collection and processing conditions should be aimed at minimizing contamination from extraneous sources such as hands, body parts, clothes, ambient air, and so forth.

Specimens should be refrigerated or frozen, as instructed, as rapidly as possible after collection.

Specimen collection teams should be given copies of these instructions and trained in their use PRIOR to the time of anticipated need.

Urine Specimen Collection Guidlines

Urine is the preferred specimen if the suspected toxicant is an inorganic chemical. It must also be collected if the toxicant is unknown. If the volume of available specimen is limited, give preference to the tube for inorganic analyses, fill it at least half-way (5 mL) before pouring any urine into the container for organic analyses. Also, if urine specimens are frozen fairly promptly after collection, and shipped to the support laboratory within 48 hours of collection, preservatives such as nitric or sulfamic acid may be added upon receipt, even for urine mercury.

Collection procedure:

1. Instruct subjects to wash hands with soap and water.
2. Instruct subjects in how to collect urine to minimize chemical contamination:
   a. The cellophane wrapping of the urine collection container should not be opened until just before voiding.
   b. The person should leave the cap in the wrapping while voiding, fill the container using clean-catch midstream collection, then recap the container immediately.
   c. The inside of the container and the cap should not come into contact with any parts of the body, clothing, or external surfaces. Exposure to air should be minimized.
   d. For children under 3 years old, pediatric collection bags may have to be used. Follow the directions accompanying the bags for collection, then carefully decant the contents of the bag into appropriate containers.
3. The specimen should be divided as follows:
   a. Gently swirl the specimen in the capped container to resuspend solids.
   b. Immediately after mixing, pour urine into the 10-mL polystyrene conical bottom centrifuge tube to the 10-mL graduation line. Then fill the 60-mL glass bottle to within approximately an inch of the top, allow-

Table 18–2. Examples of Various Chemical Toxicant Specimen Collection Protocols

TEST	SAMPLE	COLLECTION	STORAGE	SHIPMENT
Lead (inorganic)	whole blood	prescreened EDTA Vacutainer	4-8 °C	4-8 °C
Arsenic (inorganic)	urine	prescreened container, 1% nitric acid preservative	freeze	dry ice
Volatiles (organic)	whole blood	prescreened gray-top Vacutainer	4-8 °C	4-8 °C within 72 hr
PCB/DDT (organic)	serum	silicone-free Vacutainers	freeze special glass containers	dry ice
Pesticides (organic)	urine	prescreened container	freeze special glass containers	dry ice

ing an air space for expansion when the specimen freezes. Pour any remaining urine into the 10-mL polystyrene tubes. Cap all tubes immediately (stoppering and crimping aluminum seal on the Wheaton bottle), apply specimen labels, and freeze specimens as soon as possible thereafter.

COLLECTION OF SPECIMENS FOR MICROBIAL IDENTIFICATION— GENERAL INSTRUCTIONS

Universal Precautions Statement

Since medical history and examination cannot reliably identify all persons infected with the human immunodeficiency virus (HIV) and other blood-borne pathogens, "universal blood and body fluid precautions" should be used when obtaining and handling specimens of blood and certain other body fluids from all persons. Other body fluids include amniotic, pericardial, peritoneal, pleural, synovial, and cerebrospinal fluids as well as semen and vaginal secretions. In addition, any body fluids containing visible blood and body tissues should be handled as though they might be infectious.

Gloves should be worn whenever blood or the specified body fluids are handled and when phlebotomy is being performed. Barrier precautions should be used whenever appropriate to prevent skin and mucous membrane exposure during specimen acquisition and handling. If hands become soiled, gloves should be worn. Gowns should be worn if splashing or spattering of fluids is likely. If splashing of the mouth and face is possible, masks and protective eyewear are indicated. Specimens must be transported in leakproof containers.

Take care to prevent injuries when using needles, scalpels, and other sharp instruments or devices and when disposing of used, sharp instruments. Do not recap or remove needles from disposable syringes by hand, and do not bend, break, or otherwise manipulate used needles by hand. Dispose of needles and sharp equipment in puncture-resistant containers.

Additional information on universal precautions procedures is available from local/state health departments or CDC's Hospital Infections Program.

Etiologic agents should be cultivated and shipped in a medium that will protect and ensure the viability of the microorganism during transit.

Optimum containers for different groups of etiologic agents vary depending upon the agent and the distance involved in shipment. In all instances, the primary container should be of a durable material that, when properly packaged, is leakproof and can withstand the temperature and pressure variations likely to occur during air and ground shipment.

Aseptic techniques should be used when serum specimens for serology are being separated from whole blood. Contaminated serum specimens are unsuited for almost all purposes. Paired serum specimens are preferred and in many cases required. The first specimen should be obtained as soon after the onset of illness as possible and refrigerated. The second specimen should be collected 2 to 4 weeks later. The optimal interval for collecting the serum specimens will vary with different infectious diseases. Sometimes, by collecting "unmatched" paired sera, a very rapid laboratory diagnosis can be made or at least strongly supported. Simply secure blood samples from cases early in each illness and pair or "match" them with samples from appropriately chosen persons who are convalescing.

Paired serum specimens, though desirable, are difficult to obtain and are not required for serologic tests of mycotic or parasitic diseases or for syphilis. However, when neonates are being tested for congenital syphilis, serum specimens are required from the newborn and the mother. Serologic tests for neurosyphilis require serum and cerebrospinal fluid (CSF) specimens.

When whole blood is sent for isolation of certain viral, bacterial, and parasitic agents, the blood should be kept cold but not frozen prior to shipment and shipped in wet ice, not dry ice. Ice water should not be used for packing when taken directly from the ice maker or ice trays. Rather, the wet ice should be held in a container until some liquid water collects, indicating that the ice is starting to thaw.

Then the liquid may be poured off and the specimen packed with the remaining solid ice with less fear of ruining the specimen by freezing en route. Provision should be made to prevent leakage of the water as the wet ice melts and to keep this water from the specimen (a good sealed container will suffice). Be sure that the specimen is so arranged that it will not be broken by the solid ice in which it is packed. Whole blood submitted for rickettsial isolation must be packed in dry ice and shipped frozen. Because some microbial specimens require different handling procedures, be sure to check with the diagnostic laboratory prior to shipping.

Slides with tissues sections, blood films, and smears of clinical material should be dry, free of immersion oil, properly labeled, and carefully packed in a slide mailing container. If a cardboard slide mailer is the only mailer available, it should be placed in another shipping container to ensure that the slides are not broken in transit.

When in doubt about what to collect, when to collect, and how to handle specimens, consult a standard microbiology text or your support laboratory.

Appendix 18-1 lists by major category infectious diseases most commonly investigated in the field. For each disease the listings show what specimen to collect and the standard laboratory tests used for confirmation. A separate column includes any special information or instructions.

APPENDIX 18-1

Specimen Collection in Specific Diseases

AGENT OR DISEASE	SPECIMEN(S) TO COLLECT	METHOD OF CONFIRMATION OR IDENTIFICATION	COMMENTS
Bacterial diseases—general			
Brucellosis	Blood, bone, marrow or site of localization	Culture	Prolonged incubation (4–5 days) may be necessary
	Serum	Tube agglutination or EIA	2-Mercaptoethanol agglutination test distinguishes IgG from IgM antibodies and may be diag nostically useful for chronic brucellosis. *Brucella canis* infection requires specific serologic test.
Cat scratch disease	Skin biopsy Lymph node Blood Pus	Culture, PCR	
Diphtheria	Throat swab	Culture	Put swab directly into Pai slant
Haemophilus influenzae	Blood CSF Sterile site specimen	Culture	Antigen tests sensitive but culture strongly preferable.
Legionellosis	Serum Lung tissue Respiratory secretions Water Urine	IFA DFA, culture— confirm by SAT Culture Antigen detection (RIA)	Positive IFA not conclusive, culture strongly preferable
Leptospirosis	Blood Urine Serum	Culture Culture MAT	Leptospiremia occurs during first week of illness. Leptospiruria occurs after the second week of illness. Growth occurs after several days to several weeks.

Note: See Appendix 18–3 for definitions of acronyms.

(*continued*)

Specimen Collection in Specific Diseases (*continued*)

AGENT OR DISEASE	SPECIMEN(S) TO COLLECT	METHOD OF CONFIRMATION OR IDENTIFICATION	COMMENTS
Bacterial diseases—general			
Listeriosis	CSF Blood Site of infection Placenta Food	Culture, PCR	Serology neither sensitive nor specific Serotyping and subtyping indicated for epidemiologic investigation, not for confirmation or identification
Lyme disease and other borrellioses	Serum	IFA, EIA, PCR	Serology not sensitive or specific
	Blood, skin biopsy	Culture, PCR	Clinical case definition necessary Culture requires special medium
	CSF	Culture, EIA, PCR	Indicated for patients with neurologic involvement
	Synovial fluid	EIA, PCR	
Neisseria meningitidis	CSF Blood Throat Serum	Culture, serotype, latex agglutination	Serotyping and subtyping indicated for epidemiologic investigation; not for confirmation or identification
Tularemia	Blood, lymph node, sputum, lesional material	Culture, serology, DFA	Culture is difficult, requires special media
	Lymph node, lesional material	Direct fluorescent antibody test	Laboratory hazard
	Serum	Microagglutination	
Group B streptococcus	Placenta, blood	Culture, subtyping	
Plague	Blood, lymph node, lymph aspirate, sputum, lesional material	Culture	Laboratory hazard
	Lesional material, lymph node	DFA	
	Serum	Passive hemagglutination	
Psittacosis (*Chlamydia psittaci*)	Sera	CF	

Sexually transmitted bacterial/diseases

Lymphogranuloma venereum (LGV) (*C. trachomatis*)	Bubo aspirate Serum	Culture CF	Maintain at -70 °C Negative CF test rules out LGV
Genital non-LGV infection (*C. trachomatis*)	Genital swab	Culture	Maintain at -70°C in sucrose-phosphate transport medium without penicillin
Trachoma	Conjunctival swab	Culture	Maintain at -70°C in sucrose-phosphate transport medium without penicillin
Chlamydial pneumonia (*C. pneumoniae*)	Serum	IIF-IgM	Nasopharyngeal culture supports diagnosis
Syphilis	Serum	Nontreponemal/ treponemal tests, DNA and Reiter absorption, WB	Treponemal tests available for postmortem bloods
Congenital	Serum	FTA-ABS, IgM (19S) IgM EIA	Mother's and baby's serum and history requested
Neurosyphilis	CSF	FTA-ABS CSF, VDRL (CSF), WB	
	Autopsy, biopsy, lesional material	DFA-TP	Paraffin blocks, slides or fixed material acceptable; must state fixative
Gonorrhea	Heterosexual men: U(T)[a] Women: C,R,T[a] Homosexual men: U,R,T[a]	Culture: acid production from carbohydrates, enzyme substrate tests. Serologic tests: FA, coagglutination	Suspend growth from pure culture in 75% glycerol in TSB. Store at -70°C, transport on dry ice (frozen strains may be stored at -20°C for 1–2 weeks)
Chancroid	Swab from lesion	Gram strain, culture: colonial morphology and texture (catalase, porphyrin, oxidase (tetra), nitrate reductase, alkaline phosphatase	Organism dies rapidly. Transport swabs in deep rabbit blood agar and Isovitalex swabs or freeze at -70°C in defibrinated rabbits blood

[a]U = urethra, R = rectum, T = throat, C = cervix.

(continued)

Specimen Collection in Specific Diseases (*continued*)

AGENT OR DISEASE	SPECIMEN(S) TO COLLECT	METHOD OF CONFIRMATION OR IDENTIFICATION	COMMENTS
Food-borne bacterial diseases			
Bacillus cereus	Stool Food	Culture Assay for toxin	Need at least 10^5 organisms per gram of incriminated food
Campylobacter jejuni	Stool Food	Culture	Serotyping done in special circumstances
Botulism (*Clostridium botulinum*)	Stool NG aspirate Food Serum	Culture, mouse assay for toxin Culture, mouse assay for toxin Mouse assay for toxin	Call local health department ASAP if you suspect botulism
Clostridium perfringens	Stool Food	Culture Assay for toxin	Need 10^5 organisms per gram of incriminated food Serotyping is done in special cases
Escherichia coli	Stool Food Serum	Culture, serotyping, assays for toxin production and for invasiveness Assay for antitoxic antibody	Specialized testing is needed to determine if *E. coli* belongs to one of the four groups recognized as enteric pathogens
Salmonella	Stool Food	Culture, serotyping	Antibiograms are useful epidemiologic markers; plasmid profiles and phage typing are done in special circumstances
Shigella	Stool Food	Culture, serotyping	Antibiograms are useful epidemiologic markers; plasmid profiles and colicin typing are done in special circumstances
Staphylococcus aureus	Stool	Culture, phage typing	Need 10^5 organisms per gram of incriminated food or

	Food	Assay for toxin	
	Vomitus		Detection of toxin in
	Nasal swabs		implicated food (not done at CDC)
Vibrio cholerae O1	Stool, vomitus	Culture, serotype,	Cholera is the
	Food	assay for toxin production	disease caused by toxigenic *V. cholerae* O1
	Serum	Vibriocidal and antitoxic antibodies	Call the local health department ASAP if you suspect cholera
Vibrio cholerae non-O1	Stool	Culture, serotype	Serotyping is done in
	Food	Assay for toxin production	special cases
Vibrio parahemolyticus	Stool	Culture	Need 10^5 organisms
	Food	Serotyping	per gram of incriminated food
		Kanagawa testing	All enteric pathogens have been Kanagawa-positive (hemolytic on Wagatsuma agar)
Yersinia enterocolitica	Stool	Culture, serotyping	Serotyping done in
	Food		circumstances
	Serum	Assay for antibody	

Viral diseases—general

Adenovirus	Throat swab, stool, eye swab	Culture, EIA	
	Serum	HI, CF, NT, EIA, IIF	
AIDS (retroviruses)	Blood, body fluids	Culture	
	Serum	EIA, WB	
Cytomegalovirus (CMV)	Urine, throat swab	Culture	Serologic tests of limited diagnostic value
	Serum	EIA, CF, indirect hemagglutination	
Coronaviruses	Throat swab	Culture	Serologic tests of limited diagnostic value
	Serum	CF, HI, NT, EIA	
Coxsackie virus	CSF, stool swab	Culture swab, throat swab	Serologic tests of limited diagnostic value
	Serum	NT, EIA	
Epstein-Barr virus	Blood, throat swab	Culture	
	Serum	OCH, IIF	

(continued)

Specimen Collection in Specific Diseases (*continued*)

AGENT OR DISEASE	SPECIMEN(S) TO COLLECT	METHOD OF CONFIRMATION OR IDENTIFICATION	COMMENTS
Viral diseases—general			
Echoviruses	CSF, stool, rectal swab	Culture	Serologic tests of limited diagnostic value
	Serum	NT, EIA	
Hepatitis A	Blood	EIA	
	Serum	EIA	
Hepatitis B	Blood	EIA	
	Serum	EIA, RIA	
Hepatitis D (delta)	Blood	EIA	
	Serum	EIA	
Hepatitis C (parenterally transmitted non-A, non-B)	Serum	EIA, RIA	
Hepatitis E (enterically transmitted non-A, non-B)	Serum	EIA, FA	
Herpes simplex	Vesicular fluid, brain biopsy	Culture, EIA, DFA	
	Serum	EIA, CF, indirect hemagglutination	Serologic tests of limited diagnostic value
Influenza	Throat swab	Culture, EIA	
	Serum	CF, HI, EIA	
Lassa fever	Blood	Culture	Isolation of agent in lab requires biosafety level P-4 containment
	Serum	IIF, NT	
Lymphocytic choriomeningitis	Brain	Culture	
	Serum	CF, IIF, NT	
Measles	Throat swab	Culture, EIA	Serology preferred for diagnosis
	Serum	EIA, HI, CF, NT	
Mumps	Throat swab	Culture, EIA	
	Serum	HI, CF, NT, EIA	
Mycoplasma pneumonia	Throat swab, sputum	Culture	
	Serum	CF, EIA, indirect hemagglutination, IIF	
Norwalk virus	Stool	EIA, immune electron microscopy	
	Serum	EIA	

Parainfluenza	Throat swab	Culture, EIA	
	Serum	CF, HI, EIA, IIF	
Parvovirus	Blood	EIA	
	Serum	EIA, RIA	
Picornaviruses	Stool, rectal swab, throat swab	Culture	
	Serum	NT, EIA	
Polioviruses 1–3	Stool, rectal swab, throat swab, CNS tissue	Culture	
	Serum	NT, CF	
Rabies	Brain, skin biopsy	Culture, DFA	
	Serum	RFFIT, IFA	
Repiratory syncytial virus	Throat swab	Culture, EIA	
	Serum	CF, EIA, NT	
Rotavirus	Stool	EIA, culture, electron microscopy, gel electrophoresis	
	Serum	EIA, NT	
Rubella	Throat swab	Culture, EIA	Serology preferred for diagnosis
	Serum	EIA, HI, latex agglutination, IIF	
Vaccinia	Vesicular fluid, scabs, brain	Culture, electron microscopy	
	Serum	EIA, HI, NT	
Varicella zoster	Vesicular fluid	Culture, electron microscopy	
	Serum	IIF, CF	

Vector-borne viral diseases

California encephalitis	Serum	EIA, HI, CF, NT	
	Brain	Virus isolation	Except where noted, freeze specimens for virus isolation at -65 °C (dry ice)
	CSF	Virus isolation, EIA	
	Mosquitoes	Virus isolation, EIA	
Colorado tick fever	Whole blood clot	Virus isolation	Do not freeze samples for CTF virus isolation
	Serum	IIF, EIA, CF, NT	
	Ticks	Virus isolation, EIA	
Dengue 1–4	Serum	Virus isolation, HI, CF, NT, EIA, PCR	
	Liver, lung, lymph nodes	Virus isolation, antigen detection	Freeze tissues at -70°C and fix in formalin

(continued)

Specimen Collection in Specific Diseases (*continued*)

AGENT OR DISEASE	SPECIMEN(S) TO COLLECT	METHOD OF CONFIRMATION OR IDENTIFICATION	COMMENTS
Vector-borne viral diseases			
Eastern equine encephalitis	Serum	Virus isolation, HI, CF, NT, EIA, IIF	
	Brain	Virus isolation	
	CSF	Virus isolation, EIA	
	Mosquitoes	Virus isolation, EIA	
	Horse sera	HI, CF, NT, EIA	
St. Louis encephalitis	Serum	HI, CF, NT, EIA, IIF	
	Urine	EIA, virus isolation	
	Brain	Virus isolation, EIA, IIF	
	CSF	Virus isolation, EIA	
	Mosquitoes	Virus isolation, EIA	
Venezuelan equine encephalitis	Serum	Virus isolation, HI, CF, NT, EIA, IIF	Isolation requires level P-3 containment
	Brain	Virus isolation, IIF, EIA	
	CSF	Virus isolation, EIA	
	Mosquitoes	Virus isolation, EIA	
	Horse sera	Virus isolation, HI, CF, NT, EIA	
Western equine encephalitis	Serum	HI, CF, NT, EIA, IIF	
	Brain	Virus isolation, IIF, EIA	
	CSF	Virus isolation, EIA	
	Mosquitoes	Virus isolation, EIA	
	Horse sera	Virus isolation, HI, CF, NT, EIA	
Yellow fever	Serum	Virus isolation, EIA, PCR, CF, HI, NT, IIF	
	Liver	Virus isolation, histopathology, EIA	
	Mosquitoes	Virus isolation, EIA	
Rickettsial diseases			
Q fever	Serum	CF, IIF	Isolation of organisms in lab requires biosafety level P-3 containment
	Lung, blood	Culture	

Rocky Mountain spotted fever	Serum Brain, spleen, blood	IIF, Culture, DFA	Isolation of organisms in lab requires biosafety level P-3 containment
Murine typhus	Serum Blood	IIF Culture	
Ehrlichiosis	Blood, spleen Serum	Culture IIF	

Mycotic infections

Aspergillosis	Serum Tissue, site of infection	ID Histology, direct examination, culture
Candidiasis	Serum Tissue	ID, LA, EIA Histology, culture
Cryptococcosis	Serum Tissue, site of infection CSF	TA, LA Histology, FA, direct exam, culture
Histoplasmosis	Serum Tissue, site of infection Urine	ID, CF Direct exam, culture, ID (exoantigen), histology, FA Antigenuria
Nocardiosis	Serum Tissue, site of infection	ID Direct exam, culture
Sporotrichosis	Serum Tissue, site of infection	TA, LA Histology, FA, direct exam, culture

Parasitic infections

Amebiasis	Serum Tissue Formalin- and PVA-preserved stool	IHA Direct examination Trichrome stain
Cryptosporidiosis	Formalin-preserved stool Tissue Serum	Direct examination of concentrated stool stain by modified Kinyoun (acid-fast) stain or DFA Histopathology

(continued)

Specimen Collection in Specific Diseases (*continued*)

AGENT OR DISEASE	SPECIMEN(S) TO COLLECT	METHOD OF CONFIRMATION OR IDENTIFICATION	COMMENTS
Parasitic infections			
Giardiasis	Formalin-preserved stool PVA-preserved stool	Direct examination of concentrated stool or DFA	
Leishmaniasis	Serum Tissue Tissue impression smears	CF or IFA Direct exam of tissue or impression smears Culture	
Malaria	Blood smear Serum	Direct exam IIF	
Schistosomiasis	Formalin-preserved stool	Exam of concentrated stool for eggs	Tissue diagnosis occasionally necessary for diagnosis; rectal biopsy more common
	Fresh urine (examine within 45 minutes or preserve with formalin)	Examination of centrifuged urine sediment	Serologic tests helpful in acute or ectopic schisto-somiasis
Toxoplasmosis	Serum Tissue	IFA or ELISA Direct exam	IgM antibodies against *Toxoplasma* indicate recent exposure but may be detectable by EIA for 6 months to a year after infection
Trichinellosis	Serum Tissue sample of suspect meat	BF Direct exam of biopsied tissue	In addition to pork, other meats such as bear, walrus, and horsemeat have been implicated as the source of infection

APPENDIX 18-2

ABBREVIATED PROCEDURES FOR PREPARING AND SHIPPING SPECIMENS TO THE SUPPORT LABORATORY

Plan the collection schedules so that all steps required for preparing the vials for shipment can be performed within the acceptable time limits. Prepare a worklist with each specimen ID, checking off vials as prepared. If any vial cannot be filled, or if serum is hemolyzed, lipemic, or icteric, please note these comments on the worksheet. Send a xerox copy as a transmittal sheet along with the shipment to the laboratory.

Wear disposable powder-free latex or nitrile gloves during all phases of the specimen collection and processing steps. Close all vial caps tightly to prevent leakage. Make sure labels are applied neatly, going along the length of the vial or around the middle of the specimen container so that the ID can be clearly read, and the volume of the specimen can be seen. Dispose of the Vacutainer tubes properly as biohazard materials.

For frozen specimens, place labelled processed specimen vials in a rack or in a support container to allow freezing of contents with the vial in the upright position.

Supplies to be Furnished by Support Laboratory

1. Shipping containers, preferably styrofoam insulated shippers, with outer cardboard covers and lids
2. Packing material, such as plastic "bubble-pack" sheets
3. Nylon-reinforced strapping tape
4. Reusable refrigerant packs. (These must be placed in a -20°C freezer for a minimum of 2 hr before use to be hard frozen.)

Preparing Specimens for Frozen Shipments

1. Assemble shipping containers, packing materials, dry ice, paper towels or newspaper, and insulated gloves. Work quickly so that the frozen specimens will not be exposed to ambient temperatures for more than a few minutes to keep them in a hard-frozen state.
2. Place the specimens in partitioned cardboard storage boxes, or individually wrap them with bubble-pack material so that they are well cushioned.
3. Specimen shippers should be insulated styrofoam containers with outer cardboard cartons. Use either cube or "pellet" dry ice (12 lbs per ship-

per). Fill out a blank shipping list itemizing participant identification numbers, name codes, numbers of vials (or other specimen types such as tissues or foods) collected, and dates of collection and mailing for each shipment. Next to each participant's ID, neatly place one of the extra patient labels for ID verification upon receipt. Include one copy of the shipping list with the shipper under the outer lid, and fax a copy to the receiving laboratory to track shipments. Retain a third copy for your records.

4. When packing the shipment, follow these instructions:
   a. Wearing insulated gloves, put a layer of dry ice on the bottom of the shipper.
   b. Cover ice with several paper towels or sheets of newspaper.
   c. Place the boxes or bundles of bubble-wrapped specimens on the paper towels.
   d. Cover with another layer of towels.
   e. Add the rest of the dry ice (do not use styrofoam chips).
   f. Make sure the styrofoam inner lid of the shipper is completely closed to preserve dry ice life.
   g. Place the shipping list on top of the styrofoam lid, then secure the outer cardboard lid firmly with clear or nylon reinforced strapping tape, and attach the air express courier label. Indicate approximate weight of enclosed dry ice on label.

Shipments should be shipped by air express courier to the analytical laboratory you are using. Do not ship to arrive on a weekend or on a holiday, if it can be avoided, without first notifying the recipients. Send a faxed copy of the transmittal sheet so that your shipment will be anticipated and can be tracked if delayed.

Preparing Specimens for Refrigerated Shipment

Following the general instructions previously outlined for preparing specimens, place several frozen refrigerant packs on the bottom of the shipper. Place packaged specimens on top of the packs, followed by a top layer of frozen packs. This "sandwich" provides cool temperatures for up to 48 hr. Specimens to be shipped in this manner include all the Vacutainers for whole blood and non-perishable foods.

APPENDIX 18–3

LIST OF ABBREVIATIONS

BF	Bentonite flocculation
CF	Complement fixation
CSF	Cerebrospinal fluid
EIA	Enzyme immunoassay
DFA	Direct fluorescent antibody
DFA-TP	Direct fluorescent antibody for *Treponema pallidum*
ELISA	Enzyme-linked immunoabsorbent assay
FA	(Direct) fluorescent antibody
FTA-ABS	Fluorescent treponemal antibody–absorption
HI	Hemagglutination inhibition
ID	Immunodiffusion
IEP	Immune electrophoresis
IFA	Indirect fluorescent antibody test
IIF	Indirect immune fluorescence
IHA	Indirect hemagglutination
Isol.	Isolation
LA	Latex agglutination
MAT	Microscopic agglutination
NG	Nasogastric
NT	Neutralization test
OCH	Ox cell hemolysin
PCR	Polymerase chain reaction
PHA	Passive hemagglutination
PVA	Polyvinyl alcohol
Resp.	Respiratory
RFFIT	Rapid fluorescent focus inhibition test
RIA	Radioimmunoassay
SAT	Slide agglutination test
TA	Tube agglutination
VDRL	Venereal Disease Research Laboratory
WB	Western blot

INDEX